Prescription Strength

"Wherever the art of medicine is loved, there is also a love for humanity."

– Hippocrates

"The good physician treats the disease; the great physician treats the patient who has the disease."

– William Osler

"The aim of medicine is to prevent disease and prolong life; the ideal of medicine is to eliminate the need for a physician."

– William J. Mayo

"I believe that the greatest gift you can give your family and the world is a healthy you."

– Joyce Meyer

"You are not accidental. The world needs you. Without you, something will be missing in existence, and nobody can replace it."

– Rajneesh

Praise

"The science is unstoppable."

– Los Angeles Tribune

"Few things are more satisfying than seeing someone's life change through weight loss and energy gains. After all, I became a doctor to not just extend life but also to expand its quality."

– Dr. Yael Myers

"I knew I needed something stronger, and this book's treatment gave me the strength to lengthen my life."

– Sally Smith (Miami Weight Loss patient)

"I only wish I knew sooner."

– Ralph Fields

"My kids have told me for years that they were concerned for my health, but I just didn't have the knowledge or strength to really make a change until Dr. Soffer helped me."

– Peter Warren (Boca Raton Weight Loss Patient)

Praise

"This is my new Number 1 recommendation for anyone that needs to lose weight and keep it off."

– Tyler Ornstein (TylersCoffee.com)

"This book is a companion guide to our weight loss treatment."

– Dr. Furqan Tejani (Board Certified Cardiologist in NYC)

"I never realized all I could do and would do until I had the energy that came from losing the weight."

– Sarah Stone

"I read everything, I tried everything, but it wasn't until I worked with Dr. Soffer and this book that real lasting results arrived."

– Janet Jones (Hollywood Weight Loss patient)

"The cravings might be the hardest part, the mountain I couldn't climb but that all changed once a doctor prescribed what I call the craving killer. Thank you!"

– Lois Reed

Copyright

Prescription Strength: The Physicians Guide to Effortless Weight Loss

Library of Congress 2023916251

Paperback ISBN 978-1-959473-00-8

Hardback ISBN 978-1-959473-01-5

ASIN B0CHLHWHT6

SimpleMD.com

This book is intended for information purposes only. It is not intended to serve as a substitute for professional medical advice. The author and publisher assume no responsibility or liability arising directly or indirectly from the use of any of the information included in this book. This publication is not intended to diagnose, treat, or describe any specific medical condition. A qualified health professional should be consulted regarding specific medical conditions.

All rights reserved. No part of this book may be used or reproduced in any manner whatsoever without written permission except in the case of short quotations for use in articles or reviews.

PRESCRIPTION STRENGTH

The Physician's Approach to Effortless Weight Loss

A SIMPLEMD® BOOK

DR. ARIEL SOFFER

Former On-Air Medical Expert for ABC News

SimpleMD®
WEIGHT LOSS MADE SIMPLE

TOP TALENT
PUBLISHING

Table of Contents

Dedication — 1
Special Thanks — 2
Foreword — 4
Introduction — 8

PART 1 Why

Chapter 1 Why This Book — 14
Chapter 2 Why You're Stuck — 20

PART 2 How

Chapter 3 Manifest Goals — 32
Chapter 4 Modern Medications — 42
Chapter 5 Maximize Meals — 58
Chapter 6 Mindful Movements — 96

PART 3 Results

Chapter 7 More Rest — 108
Chapter 8 Monitor with Technology — 118
Chapter 9 Master Your Emotions — 126
Chapter 10 Make Healthy Habits — 134

PART 4 Teamwork

Chapter 11 Building Your Dream Team — 146
Chapter 12 Leveling Up — 154

Epilogue — 164

The SimpleMD® Manifesto — 168

Online Resources — 169

Reading List — 169

Dedication

No useful body of work is done in isolation. My 40-year journey from pre-med college to medical school, residency, fellowship, academic, and private practice has been a long road that would not have existed if it wasn't for my parents. My mother and father have consistently provided nurturing love, support, and direction.

My mother, Mina Soffer, and I actually collaborated on our first medical book together. She showed me the power of perseverance and the importance of making complex things simple.

My father, Gad Soffer, as a university professor and natural academic, helped me to be prolific and studious every step of the way with balance that includes fun and excitement.

My brother Avi and my sister Emira have always supported my efforts and been there for useful critique and helpful suggestions, love and support.

Of course, my wife, my queen, my "Malka", Ana Maria Soffer. Her eternal optimism, unconditional love and consistent way of being has allowed me to pursue my life's work. Our children Evan and Shayna have kept me driven to make the world a better place to live filled with knowledge and wisdom.

And, in remembrance of our dear family friend, Eli Silverman. Through his 19 incredible years of life his lightness of being and depth of soul will always be amongst us.

Special Thanks

Professionally this publication could not have been completed without these instrumental colleagues and friends. Our South Florida SofferHealth team starts with Tainet Gonzalez, my assistant and practice manager extraordinaire, a loyal and lovely addition to all our lives with more than two decades of dedicated service. She is family and holds a special place in our hearts.

Thanks also to our amazing nursing and support staff in South Florida including Cecilia Pernas, Lori Eduartez, Kim Eduartez, Nicolette Tabacco, Roberto Rodriguez, Mily Sartorio, Dina Bielski, Kerri Adamy, Kathleen Picardi, Daniela Gardner, Mirka Roque, Natalia Grugel, Alex Castro, and Merlyn Castillo.

Special mention to my colleague, friend and personal physician, Dr. Yael Myers whose wisdom and love is always a blessing and makes our long days in clinic seem so worthwhile. Dr Furquan Tejani, my "brother from another mother," who has recently given me the inspiration to continue to add to our life's work as cardiologists with another milestone that will hopefully continue to improve lives.

And finally, to my research, writing and content creation team including David T. Fagan, Isabel Donadio, JonVanZile, and Katerina Perez, thank you for bringing my work to the pages of a book that will hopefully continue to improve many lives for years to come.

5 THINGS TO QUIT RIGHT NOW

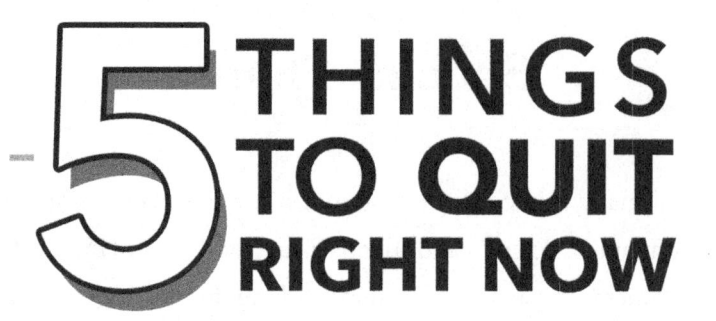

- ✗ TRYING TO PLEASE EVERYONE.
- ✗ FEARING CHANGE.
- ✗ LIVING IN THE PAST.
- ✗ PUTTING YOURSELF DOWN.
- ✗ OVERTHINKING.

Foreword

By Donald J. Waldrep, MD, FACS. Internationally recognized and Board Certified Bariatric Surgeon and Inventor of the WRAP weight loss surgery.

In the intricate world of medicine, where every decision can have profound implications on a patient's life, it is a rare privilege to come across pioneers who not only excel in their respective fields but also pave the way for others to follow. Dr. Soffer is one such luminary in the realm of cardiovascular and weight loss medicine.

I have been privileged to have known him since his early years at Cedars Sinai Medical Center/UCLA. His expertise, dedication, and relentless pursuit of excellence have not only changed and saved countless lives but have also inspired many, including myself, to push the boundaries of what's possible in our respective specialties.

The journey of weight loss, particularly when it involves medical intervention, is a complex one. It demands a holistic approach, where every aspect of a patient's individual health is taken into consideration. And it is here that Dr. Soffer's expertise becomes invaluable.

His collaborative creation of SimpleMD® stands as a testament to his vision of creating a seamless and coordinated medical journey for patients. In my years of practicing bariatric surgery and developing the WRAP bariatric technique, I have seen firsthand the challenges patients face with medical weight loss. The need for a comprehensive, coordinated care system is undeniable.

Now, with these novel groundbreaking medications, such a system is of absolute importance for patients long term success.

SimpleMD® bridges this gap, providing an ecosystem where all the stakeholders in a patients weight loss success can collaborate, ensuring that the patient's journey is not just about weight loss, but about holistic well-being.

In this book and the program that it supports, you will find a treasure trove of insights, not just about the science of weight loss, but about the art of medicine itself. It is a reflection of the dedication of professionals like Dr. Soffer and his colleagues and the commitment of companies like SimpleMD® to make the medical weight loss journey as coordinated, effective, and effortless as possible.

To Dr. Soffer, SimpleMD®, and to all the readers, I hope this book serves as a beacon of hope, knowledge, and inspiration. Here's to a healthier, brighter future for all.

-Donald J. Waldrep, MD, FACS
Beverly Hills, California

Dr. Donald J Waldrep, MD FACS, developed what has been called "a top tier bariatric surgery practice" in the United States. Innovator of "The WRAP" – the new stomach re-shaping procedure revolutionizing weight loss surgery – Dr. Waldrep has successfully helped thousands of patients in Beverly Hills and surrounding areas reach their weight loss goals.

Dr. Waldrep and his many patients have been featured on popular outlets like NBC-TV, ABC-TV, E! Entertainment, USA Today.com, Sacramento Bee, the Ventura Star, and nationally syndicated health and weight loss specials.

His experience includes:
- Fellow of the **American College of Surgeons**
- Fellow of the **American Society for Bariatric & Metabolic Surgery**
- Diplomate of the **American Board of Surgery**
- **Medical Director for a Bariatric Surgery *Center of Excellence***
- Certification by the **American Society for Metabolic & Bariatric Surgery** Essentials, Advanced, and Masters Courses
- Certificates in bariatric surgery training from the University of Pittsburgh and **Stanford University**
- Personally performed s**everal thousand laparoscopic weight-loss surgeries**, including Gastric Bypass, Gastric Banding, Gastric Sleeve and ORBERA Balloon
- First private-practice FDA sanctioned "Low BMI" Banding, revision surgeries, and now a leading experience in evaluating the role of Imbrication Gastroplasty
- Appointed as surgical expert on the **Obesity Provider Toolkit Expert Panel**; an educational consensus panel comprised of the California Medical Association Foundation (CMA Foundation) and California Association of Health Plans (CAHP). This is the first expert panel meeting to collaboratively develop an Obesity Provider Toolkit addressing the growing obesity epidemic in the state of California
- Author for several articles on advanced laparoscopic surgery and traditional general surgery in Journal of the Society of Laparoendscopic Surgeons, Annals of Surgery, American Journal of Surgery, Surgical Endoscopy, Journal of the American College of Surgeons, and American Surgeon, as well as several textbook chapters

Introduction

This book might be the most complete and comprehensive approach to weight loss. There are books about mindset, diets, exercise, and advice from doctors, but this has to be one of the best books to combine so much of all of this and more. It's the perfect combination of modern-day medicine, healthy eating, physical fitness, personal development, cutting-edge tech, and more.

With no silver bullets in health and wellness, so much of successful physical wellbeing has to do with putting all the odds in your favor. The angels are truly in the details. Not to mention there are different blood types, body types, sexes, diseases, people with various injuries, genetic coding with DNA predisposed to diseases and varying levels of active living that there needs to be room for customization.

This book addresses all of that and more in a way that allows medical professionals and various clinicians to assist you along your journey to the healthiest you possible.

Not only does this book address all the most important ways to achieve the leanest body with the longest life possible, it provides you with a roadmap to keep you on the path of perpetual health. Or, at least it puts all the odds in your favor so that you might make the most out of the body you were born into.

From the 8 Pillars of Perpetual Health to the case studies, meal recipes, exercise examples, checklists, and done for you solutions you're bound to get value. Achieving your greatest health goals have never been easier than with the advice in this book. Whether you just want to shed a few pounds as a woman or sculpt a six pack as a man, this book can help. Even if you're a man looking to lose a few pounds or a woman looking to have a six pack, it's within reach.

The secret is to start where you are, use what you have and do what you can. Before you know it, momentum is moving in your favor, habits are being formed and results are being reached. From there you can take it up a notch or hold steady at your latest accomplishment. Mind you these are my words but rather the words you will read on the pages of this book.

Although this book presents information and education that you can easily take action on in a somewhat chronological order, I noticed this book could easily be read out of order with every chapter really standing on its own. It's what we call skimmable for you "gold nugget searchers" as well as detailed for you "anal types". You know who you are.

Just don't forget that unlike a lot of fad diets from fitness influencers, this book is designed to be Prescription Strength with a physician or clinician involved in the process. As you'll read more about in this book, you will be building your dream team to reach what you thought were unreachable goals. That team requires licensed practitioners to help you limit your risks and put all the odds in your favor.

Be safe, lose weight, get healthy, and live a long life!

Enjoy!

Top Talent Publishing

> "[TO GET] *something* YOU'VE NEVER HAD, YOU HAVE <u>TO DO</u> SOMETHING YOU'VE NEVER DONE."
>
> – Unknown

PART 1
Why

ALMOST EVERY SUCCESSFUL PERSON BEGINS WITH **TWO BELIEFS**...

THE FUTURE CAN BE **BETTER** THAN THE PRESENT

——— AND ———

I HAVE THE POWER TO MAKE IT SO.

CHAPTER 1
Why This Book

Dear Reader,

There are few things more difficult than losing weight. This challenge is only compounded when you not only want to lose weight but also keep it off. According to Psychology Today, the average person tries 162 diets over their lifetime (or roughly 2 a year) and I doubt they are trying because they found something that worked.

If you're reading this then you are in good company with a great number of other people that, like yourself, have not found a way to shed the pounds and keep them from coming back. The simple truth is that most likely you didn't fail your diet as much as it failed you. I can say that as a doctor with decades of experience as well as a chronic dieter that was stuck in the loop.

As a seasoned clinical cardiologist, medical educator, and author, over time, I've refined my professional focus. I've transitioned from being just a reactive physician to one who is deeply committed to preventive care. By also aiding people in weight loss, I preemptively combat heart disease and a host of other serious medical conditions before they can take hold in the body. This shift is crucial, as many health issues stem from poor dietary choices, unhealthy habits, and the physical strain of carrying excess weight.

Presctiption Strength

In addition, we all have different weaknesses or home situations that can stack the odds against us. You may want to eat differently or better but what about the other people living in your home? After all, my friends and family may not need to eat like me to be healthy. Some people travel with limited healthy options or others work in an office scenario with limited healthy situations.

With this in mind, SimpleMD® created the 8 Pillars of Perpetual Health and Wellbeing. Although some of the topics may sound familiar, some are fairly new or modern. Plus, the complete combination of these pillars holds up something that is both special and full of potential.

The 8 Pillars of Perpetual Health and Wellbeing include:
1. Manifest Goals
2. Modern Medications
3. Maximize Meals
4. Mindful Movements
5. More Rest
6. Monitor with Tech
7. Master Your Emotions
8. Make Healthy Habits

*These are laid out in a somewhat chronological and they are not all created equal as you will learn in this book.

When you hear or read Prescription Strength you probably think of #2 Modern Medications, but the truth is that everything listed in this book are things we prescribe for people through our SimpleMD® approach. It's strong and it's specific.

Why This Book

In this book, you will not only get the healthy eating and exercise options, but you will also get an education on the medications that knowledgeable doctors can prescribe for you so that you will have the strength you need to act on the knowledge you've obtained.

As the craving slows and the consistency grows the positive forward momentum is a game changer and a real difference maker for long term weight loss. I've seen it in my patients, and I've seen it in my own mirror myself. It works!

It works so well that I've shifted my mission and life's work slightly away from just being a reactionary cardiovascular specialist to one that is hyper-focused on prevention. Of course, the truth is that as I help people lose weight, I am fighting heart disease and many other serious medical conditions before they ever even have a chance to take root in the body because so much of what ails the body comes from eating unhealthy foods, developing unhealthy habits, and carrying around excessive fat that wears and tears down the body.

Whether you are new to weight loss or tried everything and failed, this book is for you and the people you love.

Thanks to the advances in medical research and medicine, things like polio and smallpox are very rare and can be prevented. Weight loss is moving in that direction. This book's 8 Pillars will prove this to be true.

Presctiption Strength

My mission is your mission, lose the weight but my life's work doesn't have to be your life's work. This book will show you how.

Sincerely,

Dr. Ariel Soffer

www.SimpleMD.com

Why This Book

Top 10 Reasons People Listen to Dr. Ariel Soffer:

1. Completed High School at 16 and Graduated with Distinction at the University of Miami Medical School several years later.

2. Excelled at Internship and Residency at Cedars Sinai Medical Center/UCLA.

3. Harvard Business School Executive Management Program, Executive Education Program, Boston, MA.

4. Former Team Physician for the NHL's Florida Panthers.

5. Past ABC television network On Air Medical Expert having filmed segments of "Soffer's Second Opinion" for multiple years.

6. Published multiple books including the Mediterranean Diet Book as well as the Prescription Strength: The Physicians Approach to Effortless Weight Loss.

7. Guest Lecturer at multiple schools and conferences.

8. Founder of SimpleMD® an organization supporting a network of doctors in all 50 states.

9. Creator of several patents including some that launched 8 figure companies.

10. Multiple media interviews including Dr. Oz as the "leading world expert" according to Dr. Oz himself.

THINGS THAT MATTER ∩ **THINGS YOU CAN CONTROL**

↑

WHAT YOU SHOULD FOCUS ON

CHAPTER 2
Why You're Stuck

You never stood a chance. Between the high percentage of processed foods, clever advertising, endless social situations that include unhealthy foods at the center and the highly addictive nature of sugar you might as well be digging the Grand Canyon with a toothbrush. The odds are and will ever be overwhelmingly against you.

I don't write this to discourage you but rather to help you realize what you are up against so you can ultimately overcome it all.

According to research from the Gallup polling organization, the average American gets less than the recommended 7-8 hours of sleep at night starting each morning with a sleep deficit. Breakfast is a hurried affair, often consisting of bad carbs and caffeine. You work longer hours than most people in the world with increased stress and unhealthy options eating, working, and living.

Even if you work for yourself or work from home you are still likely to have limited healthy options with maybe even less movement to burn calories.

Portion Control is Out of Control

According to the US Department of Agriculture in a study "Profiling Food Consumption in America," the average American adult consumed more than 2700 calories a day which 35% more than the recommended 2000 calories a day for an adult man. This is a whopping 24.5% increase from 1970.

Presctiption Strength

Meanwhile, according to the Centers for Disease Control and Prevention, as many as 80% of Americans don't get the recommended amount of exercise to maintain good health. If that wasn't bad enough, restaurant delivery services have exploded, allowing the unhealthiest options to become the easiest option.

Your Greatest Addiction

You're even more stuck than you might consciously realize because so much of what you consume is addictive. This isn't limited to caffeine and sugar with most simple carbs quickly turning to sugar cravings. Even salt or the need for salt is a very real thing.

Trying to cut down on caffeine can lead to bad headaches and drops in energy. Some studies have suggested that sugar is as addictive as cocaine. Whether true or not, sugar cravings are real! Your willpower and discipline have to be even stronger (some believe impossibly superhuman) when considering limiting some of these things let alone kicking them altogether.

A Vicious Cycle

You don't sleep well so you want caffeine and sugar to get going and feel well but that leads to energy crashes that keep you from exercising which leads to poor sleep and then the cycle starts all over again. At some point you have to become sick and tired of being sick and tired. At some point you have to want health, strength and energy more than a buzz or to be socially in alignment with what's happening in the moment. It's not easy!

Why You're Stuck

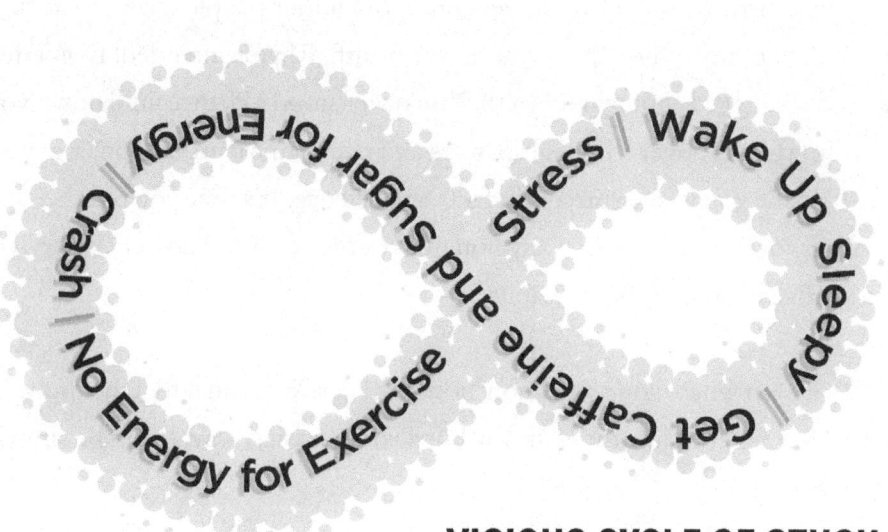

Stress | Wake Up Sleepy | Get Caffeine and Sugar for Energy | Crash | No Energy for Exercise

VICIOUS CYCLE OF STUCK

The Attraction of Easy Answers

Then you try the sexiest thing you see. You try the fad diets and one-size-fits-all ways of eating. No surprise that they didn't work or weren't sustainable. You didn't fail at your diet rather your diet failed you.

Fast Fad Answers that have You Falling Backwards may include:
- Cutting carbs without understanding simple carbs vs complex carbs
- Cutting calories and starving yourself in a way that your body works harder to store fat
- Eating a "healthy" food in excess defeating the point of the healthy food in the first place
- Exercising wrong to the point of an injury which then keeps you from exercising consistently
- Making yourself sick while eating too little and exercising too much causing you to give up

Presctiption Strength

Most of these so-called answers are more about people trying to acquire wealth than trying to help you acquire true health. Rhyme intended! Don't' feel bad or discouraged about your health. You never stood a chance until now. Now is the time to start over with real answers and real medical professionals at your side. It's time you were armed with facts and science. It's time you put the odds in your favor. It's time to shed any potential victimhood and become a survivor of addictive eating foods and habits.

I've been where you are. I know how hard it is. We're in it together now. I'll be showing you not just the best way but also the easiest way. It can be simpler than you think.

> *"When science collides with common sense, the explosion is magical. Food is cheaper now by a long way, more abundantly available, more highly refined and processed and marketed to us by very clever advertising companies and techniques. The remarkable thing is [not that we are overweight] but how anybody stays thin."*
>
> **– Andrew Prentice, Ph.D., Professor of International Nutrition, London School of Hygiene and Tropical Medicine**

Up to 70% of Americans are considered overweight or obese. This rise in obesity has become a national disaster, and to make it worse, it seems like we refuse to recognize what's really going on. Instead of trying to understand obesity as a complex metabolic disorder, we treat it like a personal failing. Not too long ago, I saw television host Bill Maher talking about the new weight loss drugs. His position—as someone who clearly is not afflicted with obesity—was that no one should have to use drugs to lose weight. Instead, they can "stop eating donuts."

Why You're Stuck

The Willpower Myth

There's so much wrong with this statement (lots of people who eat donuts aren't obese at all, and plenty of obese people would never get near a donut), but the worst part of it is the shame. This view of obesity, which goes much deeper than one talk show host, blames the people who suffer from it. According to this, obese people lack willpower. They aren't strong enough to do the "right" thing and just watch what they eat. Instead, they are gluttons, stuffing themselves with terrible foods with no regard for their health. Of course, this is ridiculous. The Wall Street Journal recently wrote an article titled Ozempic Settles the Obesity Debate: It's Biology Over Willpower. So true!

I'm sure you know plenty of people who are carrying extra weight but who exercise regularly and eat a healthy diet, just as I'm sure you know people who are very thin but who never exercise and eat whatever they want. In my own house, my wife and I have two children who were born eighteen months apart. They grew up in an identical environment but both have very different metabolic set points. The same is true for my wife and me. She's naturally thin, while I have to be much more careful.

Superstition vs. Science

In fact, most of our national discussion on weight and weight loss is terribly misguided and relies more on emotion and superstition than science. In reality, everybody has a natural set point weight. This set point is the natural weight your body wants to maintain. Your set point is mostly genetic, but it's also influenced by your environment. When people describe having difficulty losing weight or "yo-yo" dieting, it's usually because they didn't actually alter their set point.

Presciption Strength

Instead, they made a temporary change to their lifestyle patterns that resulted in weight loss, but as soon as the "diet" was over, they went back to their normal patterns and their body quickly re-established its preferred set point.

Achieving True Change

The SimpleMD® program is based on the idea that we can effectively and permanently alter our set points by making lasting changes in our lifestyles. It's not easy, but we know that it's possible to alter a set point, and once changed, it can bring a permanent change in your life.

Put simply, your set point describes the complex interplay of genetics, metabolism, and environment that governs how much your body wants to naturally weigh. It should come as no surprise that everyone is different, and we all have different set points. Studies have shown that obesity has a strong genetic component, with up to 80 percent of the variation in body weight being attributed to genetics.

The World Working Against You

The key, however, is to understand that your set point isn't your destiny. In fact, we've created an environment that seems perfectly designed to sabotage us. Even if the environment only accounts for 20 percent of our natural set point, it is a vital 20 percent. Modern society is characterized by an abundance of high-calorie, high-fat, and highly processed foods, as well as a sedentary lifestyle. These factors make it difficult for individuals to maintain a healthy weight and they contribute to the development of obesity.

Our SimpleMD® program was designed to get you unstuck. With this in mind, SimpleMD® created the 8 Pillars of Perpetual Health and Wellbeing. Although some of the topics may sound familiar some are fairly new or modern. Plus, the complete combination of these pillars holds up something that is both special and full of potential.

The 8 Pillars of Perpetual Health and Wellbeing include:
1. Manifest Goals
2. Modern Medications
3. Maximize Meals
4. Mindful Movements
5. More Rest
6. Monitor with Tech
7. Master Your Emotions
8. Make Healthy Habits

These 8 Pillars are what we prescribe and together they can't help but get healthy results. It's Prescription Strength, the strongest solution in the world today. Chapter 2 on Modern Medications is the most relevant and advanced way to lose weight making it the most important chapter you can read and advice for you to take action on. Although Chapter 3 on eating right, is the single most beneficial thing you can do when it comes to losing weight, it's the FDA Approved medications (GLP-1's) in Chapter 2 that will make eating right possible by removing your unhealthy cravings (among other benefits). As in my personal situation, these medications, combined with the other pillars, have the capacity to change your relationship with food for the better forever!

8 PILLARS OF PERPETUAL HEALTH AND WELL BEING

Maximize Meals • Modern Medications • Mindful Movements • Make Healthy Habits • Master Emotions • Monitor With Tech • More Rest • Manifest Goals

> **"DON'T LIMIT YOUR CHALLENGES**
>
> ---
>
> **CHALLENGE YOUR LIMITS."**
>
> *- Unknown*

PART 2
How

GOALS SO BIG YOU GET *Uncomfortable* TELLING SMALL MINDED PEOPLE

CHAPTER 3
Manifest Goals

It's important to have goals. In the beginning they can be simple and general but as time goes on the more specific you can make them the more likely you are to have a higher level of success. When you first start, we just want you to get some wins and from those wins we want you to gain positive forward momentum.

The most common health goal is to simply lose weight and there is nothing wrong with that! Still, if your goal is to run a marathon or to have a six pack someday your daily decisions will need to reflect that level of commitment. Just because you might have extreme goals doesn't necessarily mean you'll need extreme effort, but you will need to declare those goals in a very intentional way.

Goal setting is a lifelong process used by super successful people in business, athletics and more. Quite simply, people do it because it works.

The best goals that are most likely to be reached include 3 crucial components as outlined in the visual aid.

The 3 Components of Successful Healthy Goal Setting are:
1. Specific – You must define the goal with details.

2. Possible – You must make sure it can be done.

3. Deadline – You must have a finish line date.

HEALTHY GOAL SETTING

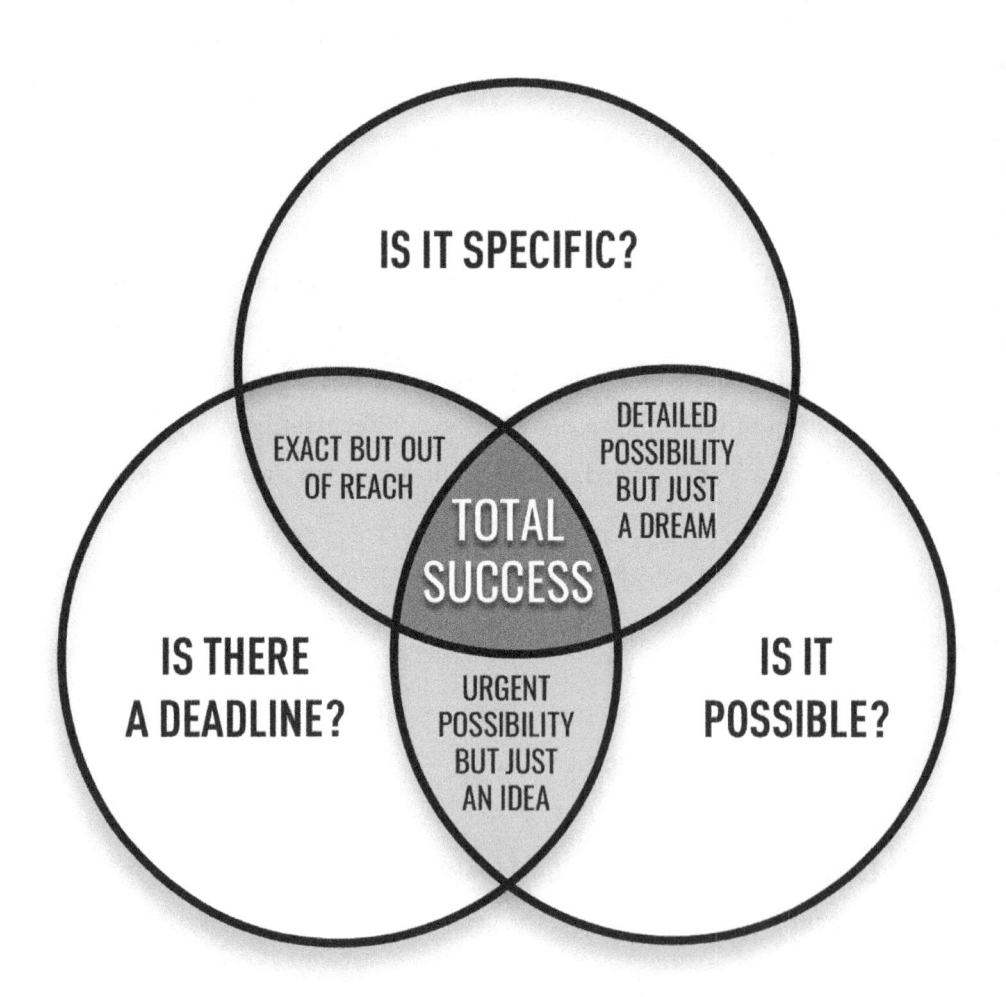

- IS IT SPECIFIC?
- IS THERE A DEADLINE?
- IS IT POSSIBLE?

- EXACT BUT OUT OF REACH
- DETAILED POSSIBILITY BUT JUST A DREAM
- URGENT POSSIBILITY BUT JUST AN IDEA

TOTAL SUCCESS

Notice the Venn Diagram, where it shows them overlapping illustrating where the goal is most likely to happen as well as what it looks like if and when you are missing one of the elements. This is about playing the odds and putting all the odds in your favor for success. This is a SimpleMD® book and the SimpleMD® practice is a full-service concierge health program with a team approach to weight loss and wellness.

SimpleMD® has a whole team (supporting clinicians all over the country) to assist you in setting your health goals as well as achieving them! Don't forget to visit SimpleMD.com to get even more detailed and up-to-date information.

The Law and Power of Accountability

We'll discuss this more in the chapter on teambuilding but suffice to say goals are drastically more like to be reached when you have someone holding you accountable. It's also best for it not to be a partner because when one falls short they lose their power and credibility to require the other person to be accountable. This marks the beginning of the end. The best people to hold you accountable are not partners, family members, or anyone that you have an equal footing.

A study by the Association for Talent Development found that individuals have the following probabilities of completing a goal by taking these actions:

1. Having an idea or goal - 10% likely to complete the goal

2. Consciously deciding that you will do it - 25% likely to complete the goal

3. Deciding when you will do it - 40% likely to complete the goal

4. Planning how to do it - 50% likely to complete the goal

Presctiption Strength

5. Committing to someone that you will do it - 65% likely to complete the goal

6. Having a person holding them accountable - 95% likely to complete the goal

The Triangle of Accountability is Most Likely to Yield Results:

TRIANGLE OF ACCOUNTABILITY

```
                    A
           C HOLDS A ACCOUNTABLE
                A HOLDS B ACCOUNTABLE
              ONE WAY
           ACCOUNTABILITY
        C                              B
           B HOLDS C ACCOUNTABLE
```

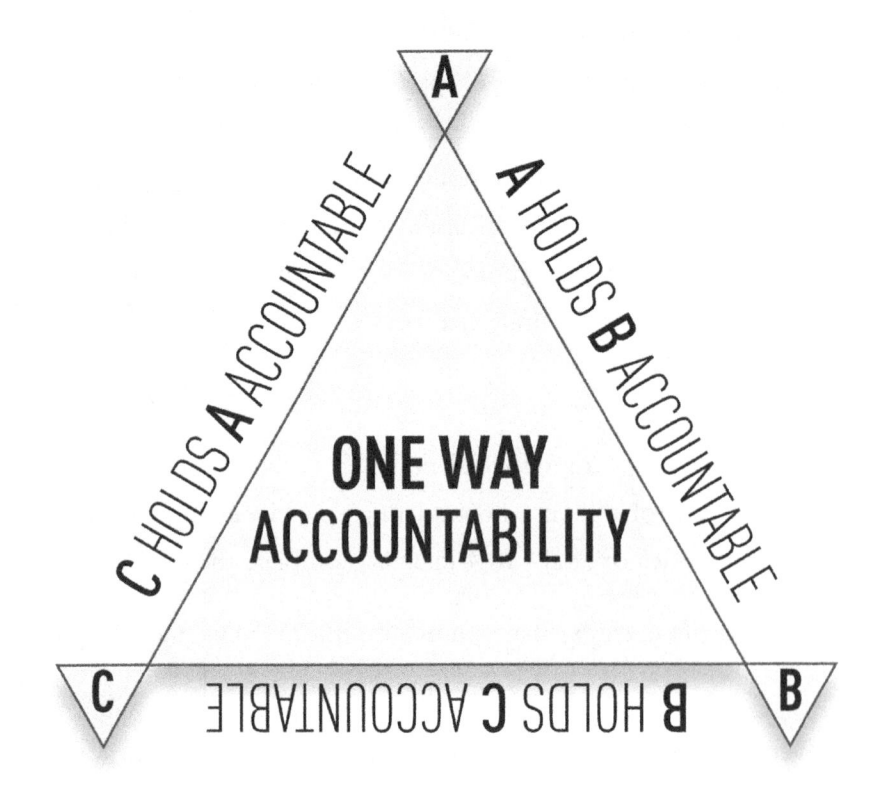

Manifest Goals

Examples of Different Ways to Quantify Your Goals

MAKING IT POSSIBLE

01 REALISTIC

02 DONE BEFORE

03 SUSTAINABLE

Presciption Strength

Deadlines of Goals might look like:

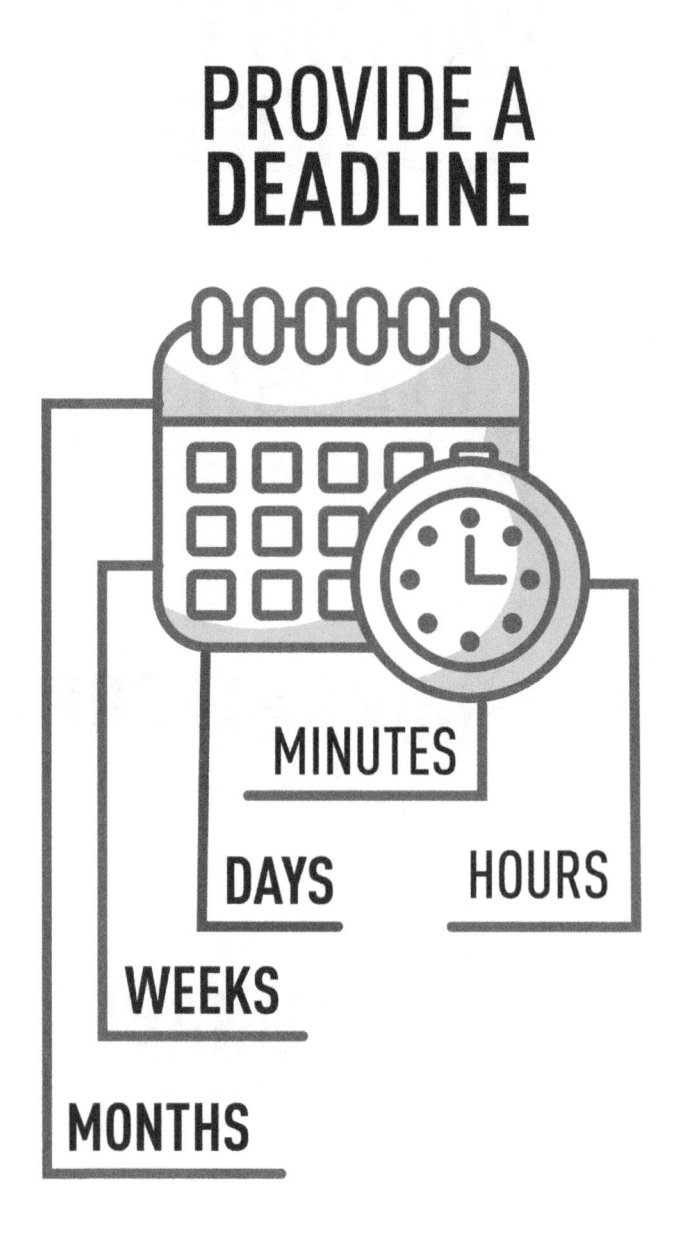

PROVIDE A DEADLINE

- MINUTES
- HOURS
- DAYS
- WEEKS
- MONTHS

Manifest Goals

Specific Goals could be related to:

SPECIFIC GOALS

- WEIGHT
- INCHES
- BODY FAT
- BLOOD PRESSURE
- MUSCLE TONE
- FLATTEN STOMACH
- ENERGY LEVEL

Presctiption Strength

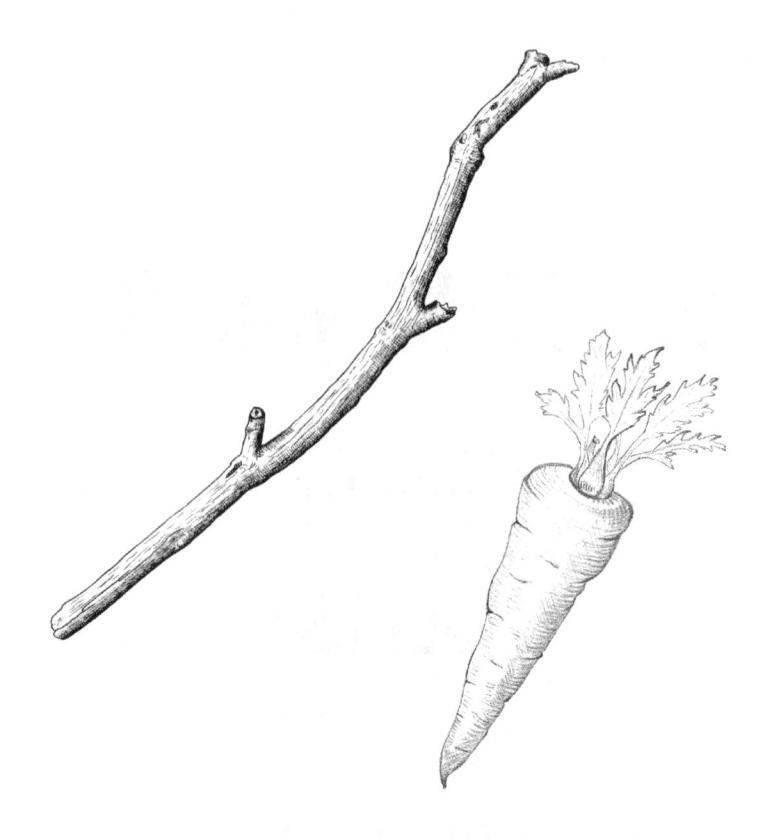

Another way to increase the likelihood of you reaching your goals are to use the carrot vs the stick method where you choose either a positive reward or a negative punishment depending on whether or not you reach the goal. Do just the carrot or just the stick or you can even use both. Learn how you're wired and how to push your buttons to drive yourself across the finish line of your ultimate goals.

Regardless of your goals, know you should have them. Even if they are small and general in the beginning have something that will give you something to work towards and measure your progress with. Making progress is important. Seeing your progress is paramount.

> "Who you've **BEEN** ISN'T WHO YOU HAVE **TO BE.**"
>
> – Unknown

> "Ozempic settles the obesity debate. It's biology over willpower. Weight-loss drugs affect the brain in ways that help researchers understand how to regulate the body."
>
> — WALL STREET JOURNAL

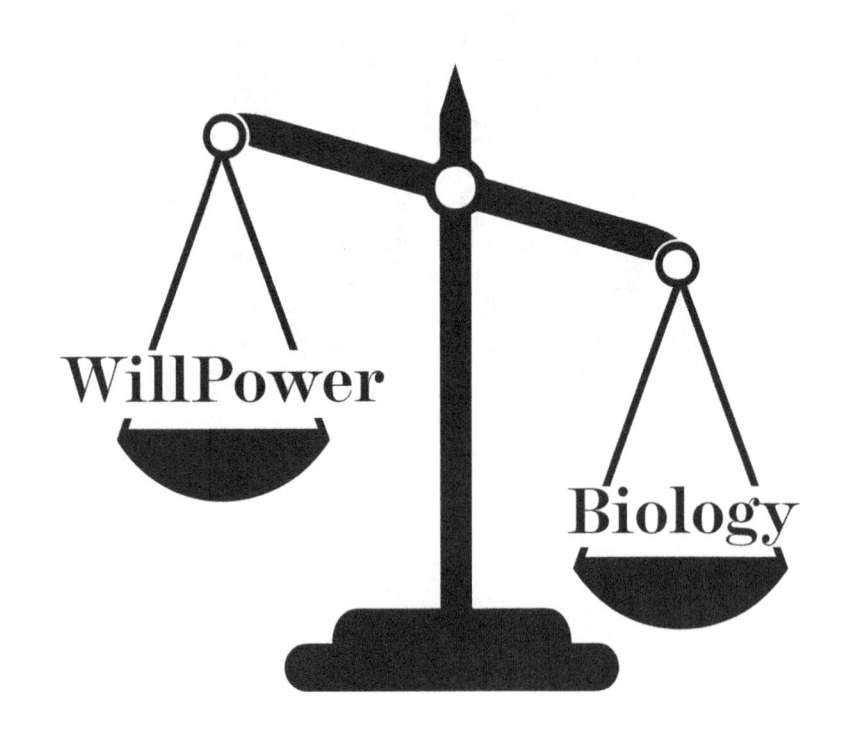

WillPower

Biology

CHAPTER 4
Modern Medications

Following this SimpleMD® program can easily result in noticeable weight loss in weeks not months. This is the start of your "reset" changing your individual weight set point on a molecular level. This sets into motion so many health benefits and even augments future capacity to lose even more weight.

We all have different weaknesses or home situations that can stack the odds against us. You may want to eat differently or better but what about the other people living in your home? After all, my friends and family may not need to eat like me to be healthy. Some people travel with limited healthy options or others work in an office scenario with limited healthy situations.

The FDA Approved Answer

We want to stop the cravings and start the consistency. Easier said than done right? Actually, now days it's never been easier with a medical professional guiding you through proven weight loss medications that will do exactly that. Imagine a world where you no longer crave the killer food and drinks. Imagine a day that you can get through without so much hunger on the brain. It's possible thanks to new FDA approved medicines called GLP-1 (which stands for Glucagon-like Peptide 1) that are used to treat diabetes mellitus and obesity.

Presctiption Strength

History and Path to Approval

GLP-1 (Glucagon-like Peptide-1) medications like semaglutide or tirzepatide are both important players in the field of weight loss drugs and medications. They work by targeting the body's natural processes to help control appetite, reduce food intake, and promote weight loss.

Here's an explanation and description:

GLP-1 is a hormone produced naturally in the gut in response to food intake. Its primary role is to regulate glucose (sugar) metabolism by stimulating insulin secretion and reducing glucagon release, both of which help lower blood sugar levels. Additionally, GLP-1 slows down gastric emptying, which leads to a feeling of fullness and reduced appetite.

Originally, weight loss medications based on GLP-1 receptor agonists, such as liraglutide and exenatide, have been developed to mimic the effects of this hormone. They are usually prescribed for individuals with type 2 diabetes, but they have also shown effectiveness in promoting weight loss in people without diabetes.

Key effects of GLP-1-based weight loss medications:
- Increased insulin secretion: Helps regulate blood sugar levels and reduces insulin resistance.
- Reduced appetite: Delays gastric emptying and promotes a feeling of fullness, leading to decreased food intake.
- Weight loss: By targeting appetite and promoting satiety, GLP-1 medications can contribute to sustained weight loss.

Modern Medications

Injected

In the context of weight loss, semaglutide or tirzepatide is typically administered as an injectable medication, often on a weekly basis. Pill or capsule based versions are also under investigation. Similar to some of the newer cholesterol medications that require only one simple injection every few months, GLP-1 injections seem very well tolerated and many patients prefer them to the daily pill delivery system. These injections have shown promising results in clinical trials, demonstrating significant weight loss in individuals who are overweight or obese, even those without type 2 diabetes.

Key effects of semaglutide or tirzepatide as a weight loss medication:
- Appetite suppression: Activates GLP-1 receptors in the brain, leading to reduced hunger and cravings.
- Weight loss: Helps individuals lose a substantial amount of weight by decreasing calorie intake and increasing feelings of fullness.

It's important to note that GLP-1-based medications, are typically prescribed under medical supervision and as part of a comprehensive weight loss plan that includes dietary changes and increased physical activity. As with any medication, they may also have potential side effects and interactions that should be discussed with a healthcare provider.

In summary, GLP-1 receptor agonists like semaglutide and tirzepatide (with many more being investigated currently) are important components of the novel weight loss medications. They work by harnessing the body's natural mechanisms to regulate appetite, control food intake, and promote weight loss, making them valuable tools in the management of obesity and related health conditions.

Presctiption Strength

Decades of Research

The history of research gathering for GLP-1 receptor agonists like semaglutide spans several decades and involves a combination of scientific discoveries, experimentation, and clinical trials. Here's an overview of the key milestones in the research and development of GLP-1 receptor agonists.

GLP-1 (Glucagon-like Peptide-1):

Discovery of GLP-1 was first discovered as a product of proglucagon gene expression in the early 1980s. Researchers identified its role in regulating glucose metabolism and its potential to stimulate insulin secretion while inhibiting glucagon release, leading to improved blood sugar control.

Quiet the Food Noise

Identification of Appetite-Regulating Effects revealed that GLP-1 played a significant role in appetite regulation. Studies demonstrated that GLP-1 administration could delay gastric emptying and induce feelings of fullness, making it a potential target for weight loss interventions.

Development of GLP-1 receptor antagonist has pharmaceutical companies develop synthetic compounds in the 2000s that mimicked the effects of GLP-1. These compounds, known as GLP-1 receptor agonists, were designed to resist degradation by enzymes in the body and provide a more sustained and effective response.

Modern Medications

Clinical Trials and FDA Approval (2000s-2010s):

GLP-1 receptor agonists such as exenatide and liraglutide were subjected to extensive clinical trials to evaluate their safety and efficacy in treating type 2 diabetes. These trials revealed not only improvements in glucose control but also significant weight loss as a side effect. The FDA approved several GLP-1 agonists for diabetes treatment.

Semaglutide:

Synthesis of semaglutide is a modified version of native GLP-1, designed to have a longer half-life in the body. This modification allows for less frequent dosing, making it more convenient for patients. Novo Nordisk, a pharmaceutical company, developed semaglutide as a potential treatment for type 2 diabetes and obesity.

Clinical Trials for Diabetes and Obesity happened in the 2010s when Semaglutide underwent rigorous clinical trials to assess its efficacy and safety for managing diabetes and obesity. It demonstrated superior glucose control and significant weight loss in individuals with type 2 diabetes. Later trials focused specifically on its potential as a weight loss medication in individuals without diabetes.

In 2021, semaglutide (branded as Wegovy®) received FDA approval as a treatment for chronic weight management in adults with obesity or overweight individuals with at least one weight-related comorbidity. It marked a significant milestone in the field of obesity treatment and offered a new tool for healthcare providers to address the obesity epidemic. In 2021-2023, The New England Journal of Medicine, considered the most prestigious medical journal by most clinicians, published a series of landmark studies on both semaglutide and tirzepatide.

Presctiption Strength

These readily available studies lead the way for many physicians to begin feeling comfortable about the risk/benefit ratio in prescribing these novel medications for their overweight and at risk patients. This scientific breakthrough led to a global shortage of these medications, the likes of which few of us in the field have ever seen.

Clinical Trials Complete

Throughout the history of research gathering for GLP-1 and semaglutide, scientific understanding of these compounds' mechanisms of action, safety profiles, and potential benefits has evolved. Clinical trials have played a crucial role in establishing their effectiveness and guiding their use in both diabetes management and weight loss interventions. Ongoing research continues to explore new applications and optimize the use of GLP-1-based medications like semaglutide for various health conditions.

In this book you will not only get the healthy eating and exercise options, but you will also get an education on the medications that knowledgeable doctors can prescribe for you so that you will have the strength you need to act on the knowledge you've obtained.

As the craving slows and the consistency grows the positive forward momentum is a game changer and a real difference maker for long term weight loss. I've seen it in my patients, and I've seen it in my own mirror myself. It works!

Modern Medications

I introduced these medications as a game-changer in the science of weight loss and healthy living. Originally touted as a way to improve blood sugar levels in diabetics, the GLP-1 medications target levels of the hormone known as glucagon-peptide 1. After researchers observed startling weight loss in study subjects, they started to focus on what was going on with these medications, and over a few years, they received FDA approval to use GLP-1 agonists for weight loss, particularly for people who had trouble losing weight The GLP-1 agonists made it possible for people to change their set point, or the natural weight their body seeks to maintain, opening up the door for long-term, sustainable weight loss.

The Science Behind the Medication

If you've been exposed to the news of these medications, you might have seen conflicting or confusing information. On the one hand, there are weight loss doctors and celebrities talking about how effective these medications are. On the other hand, there are some lifestyle celebrities and nutritionists cautioning against their use. Which is true?

In a way, both are true. GLP-1 agonists are the most powerful weight loss tool I've encountered, but they aren't a magic bullet. Lifestyle changes and improved eating are a core part of my program and the only way to achieve permanent weight loss. It's true that if you take medication for a few weeks and change nothing else, you will likely lose weight only to gain it back. I'm not recommending this kind of weight loss.

Presctiption Strength

But on the other hand, there is undeniably high-quality science demonstrating just how effective GLP-1 agonists are, even when compared to highly effective weight loss strategies like bariatric surgery.

The Exact Process of FDA Approval

The process for any drug to become FDA approved in the United States is a comprehensive and multi-phase journey that involves rigorous testing, evaluation, and regulatory scrutiny. The goal of this process is to ensure that drugs are safe and effective for their intended use before they can be sold to the general public. Here's an overview of the typical steps involved.

Preclinical Research and Development:

This stage involves laboratory research and animal testing to gather preliminary data on the drug's safety, potential efficacy, and mechanisms of action. Researchers work to identify the most promising drug candidates and assess their potential risks and benefits.

Investigational New Drug (IND) Application:

Before testing a new drug in humans, the drug's sponsor (typically a pharmaceutical company) submits an IND application to the FDA. The IND provides detailed information about the drug's composition, manufacturing process, preclinical data, and proposed clinical trial plans. If the FDA reviews the IND and raises no objections, the sponsor can proceed with conducting clinical trials.

Modern Medications

Clinical Trials (Phases I-IV) are conducted in three phases:
Phase I Small-scale trials to assess safety, dosage, and initial efficacy in a small group of healthy volunteers.
Phase II Larger trials involving patients to further evaluate safety, dosing, and efficacy, often in comparison to existing treatments.
Phase III Large-scale trials with a larger patient population to confirm safety, efficacy, and monitor side effects over an extended period.

These trials are typically randomized, double-blind, and placebo-controlled to minimize bias and provide reliable data.

New Drug Application (NDA) Submission:
After successful completion of Phase III trials, the drug sponsor submits an NDA to the FDA. The NDA includes comprehensive data from preclinical studies, clinical trials, manufacturing details, labeling, and proposed use of the drug.

FDA Review and Evaluation:
The FDA reviews the NDA to assess the drug's safety, efficacy, and overall benefit-risk profile. A team of experts evaluates the data and may request additional information or clarification. The FDA may convene advisory committees comprising external experts to provide independent opinions.

FDA Decision:
Based on the review, the FDA makes a decision on whether to approve the drug for marketing. If approved, the FDA specifies the drug's approved uses, dosages, labeling, and any necessary risk management strategies.

Presctiption Strength

Phase IV After approval and commercialization, Phase IV studies may be conducted to monitor the drug's long-term safety and real-world effectiveness. The FDA continues to monitor adverse events and can take regulatory action if new safety concerns arise.

The timeline for FDA approval can vary widely based on the complexity of the drug, the nature of the disease being treated, and the availability of data. It typically takes several years, often more than a decade, from the initial discovery to final FDA approval. However, the FDA may expedite the process for certain drugs through programs like Fast Track, Breakthrough Therapy, or Priority Review.

Once the FDA approves a drug, it can be sold to the general public for its approved indications. However, ongoing monitoring and reporting of adverse events continue to ensure patient safety.

Dealing With Side Effects

Most gastrointestinal side effects can be reduced by over-the-counter medications like Gas-X, Pepto-Bismol, or Mylanta.

- <u>Mild Nausea or Bloating</u> - This is the most common gastrointestinal side effect. It's often seen in the very beginning and during dose escalation, but for most people, it gets less significant as time passes. Studies have shown that it's caused by delayed stomach emptying, which might also mean the program is working. Some patients find this motivating, and it helps them understand the limitations of certain foods and portion sizes.

Modern Medications

- <u>GERD-Heartburn-Reflux</u> - There is a transient worsening or new onset of gastroesophageal reflux disease (GERD, a known complication of obesity) during treatment for many patients. Medications such as proton-pump inhibitors or H2-blockers can be used on a temporary basis. Possible treatment can be with omeprazole (Prilosec, once or even twice a day); for breakthrough pain, H2-blockers such as Pepcid AC, Tagamet, Protonix, and Prevacid could be used. Consult your clinician to see what might be best for you.

- <u>Constipation</u> - This is a common side effect due to the medication or, even more likely, the change of food. Treatment includes fiber supplements such as Metamucil capsules two or three times a day with several glasses of water, stool softeners, and/ or Miralax. I personally try to use a packet every morning of the Metamucil Sugar Free Orange in 6-8 ounces of cool water. It not only tastes good, but it also helps fulfill my water intake, improves fullness, and is good for my colon.

- <u>Vomiting</u> - This less common side effect usually occurs in the initial phase rather than with higher doses. Treatment for GERD-like symptoms can usually stop the vomiting.

- <u>Pancreatitis, Gallbladder Disease</u> - Both these medical problems are relatively uncommon but much more serious than the nonspecific symptoms due to gastric motility or GERD. Both consist of severe, recurrent pain, often going to the back. Anyone with severe pain needs to be fully evaluated, potentially including laboratory tests and/or diagnostic imaging. Obviously, the GLP-1s should be discontinued and not restarted if pancreatitis is found.

Presctiption Strength

Linking the Mediterranean Lifestyle

First came a 2020 European landmark study in which Dr. Antonio Di Mauro and his colleagues published a randomized controlled clinical trial in a peer-reviewed medical journal showing that levels of GLP-1 increased in patients following the Mediterranean Lifestyle when compared with those following even a vegetarian nutritional regimen (previously thought to be even healthier). This was important because it linked the Mediterranean Lifestyle to GLP-1 levels and was a building block in understanding how GLP-1 works.

My Personal Praise

Not surprisingly, in 2021, another publication stated that the Mediterranean Lifestyle, along with the novel GLP-1 medications, had the greatest effect ever seen when it comes to weight control.

Feeling fuller and boosting metabolism by affecting the weight control centers of the brain was now possible—and I can personally confirm the results in our patients (and myself) have been amazing!

They both work in part, it seems, by manipulating the level of the hormone glucagon-like peptide 1. GLP-1s are powerful hormones made by the intestinal system that sends signals to your brain to regulate your metabolism, reduce your appetite, and help you feel full. Previous studies suggest that people who hold onto more weight experience reductions in GLP-1 signaling.

Thus, it was hypothesized that amplifying those signals might help patients to easily lose more weight. GLP-1s work by counteracting the normal hunger and increased appetite that occur when you begin to lose weight and your body struggles to maintain your set point. They improve overall metabolism and overall health. From a weight-loss perspective, at least in our clinic, they've enabled patients to lose significant weight and keep it off.

We have many patients who've experienced sustained weight loss even after the medications are stopped. Our clinicians truly believe that the combination effect of the GLP-1s and the Mediterranean Lifestyle combine to help patients achieve their desired long-term results in weight loss while also reducing inflammation and insulin resistance, improving cholesterol, and reducing waist circumference.

Imagine a Life with Less Medications

If you have existing conditions (such as arthritis, high blood pressure, or diabetes), you'll likely notice improvements there, and you may even be able to reduce or stop some medications.

There are many new medications on the market today with more coming. Semaglutide seems to be the most studied medication in this category so far, with tirzepatide emerging right behind it. Tirzepatide is a glucose-dependent insulinotropic polypeptide, or hormone, that works by a somewhat different mechanism but affects the GLP-1 receptor as well.

Brand Name Medications

Rather than spend time going over each of these hormones' molecules and their various branded forms, suffice it to say that this category of medications and their associated once-per-week subcutaneous injection capacity have completely changed our ability to obtain significant weight loss. Whether it is with Wegovy, Ozempic, Mounjaro, Saxenda, Rybelsus, or any of the existing or upcoming medications in these categories, when combined with the fundamentals of the

Presciption Strength

Mediterranean Lifestyle, we expect patients to experience both short- and long-term benefits and make significant changes.

Organizations like SimpleMD® are dedicated to trying to "declutter" all the confusion around which weight loss medication might be best for which patient, how much and how long should they be taken, what side effects to be wary of, and how to best afford them. SimpleMD® accepts no remuneration from any pharmaceutical company, and its basic mission is to support patients and clinicians in trying to find the best long term weight loss solution for each individual patient.

Emma Pushes Past Her Plateau

Emma has been making remarkable progress on her weight loss journey with the help of SimpleMD®, an invaluable resource providing her with a supportive healthcare team and innovative treatment options. However, she soon encountered an unexpected obstacle—a plateau that threatened to dampen her spirits. Little did she know that a simple change and the unwavering support of her SimpleMD® team would propel her forward to achieve her ultimate goal.

Emma had diligently followed her prescribed treatment plan, which included the use of GLP-1 injections. These injections had been instrumental in her weight loss progress, but as her body adapted to the treatment, she found herself at a standstill. Frustration settled in as she desperately sought a solution to break through the plateau and continue her journey toward her goal.

Feeling disheartened, Emma reached out to her SimpleMD® team for guidance. Recognizing the significance of her struggle, they carefully reviewed her progress and discussed potential adjustments to her treatment. After thoughtful consideration, Emma's healthcare team suggested a simple change that could make a significant difference—altering her injection site from her abdomen to her shoulder.

With newfound hope, Emma embraced the change wholeheartedly. She found comfort in the guidance and support provided by her SimpleMD® team, knowing that she was not alone in her journey. Emma powered through her plateau, injecting the GLP-1 medication into her shoulder with renewed determination.

Days turned into weeks, and Emma's perseverance paid off. The plateau that had once seemed insurmountable gradually crumbled before her eyes. The weight she had been striving to shed began to melt away once again as if the change in injection site had reignited her body's response to the treatment.

Emma's confidence soared as she witnessed her progress. The support and encouragement to persevere from her SimpleMD® team and the change in the injection site fueled her motivation to reach her goal. Her commitment to her health never wavered, and her determination to overcome obstacles grew stronger each day.

Four weeks later, Emma stood before the mirror, her heart filled with pride and joy. She had surpassed the plateau, lost the remaining weight, and achieved her ultimate goal. It was a moment of triumph, a testament to her resilience and the unwavering support she had received from SimpleMD®.

CHOICES

ARE THE HINGES OF DESTINY.

EDWIN MARKHAM

CHAPTER 5
Maximize Meals

There might not be anything more important than eating right. If you wanted to knock over the biggest and best first domino that's most likely to knock over every other health goal domino you ever had in the past, and can dream up in the future, it would be to eat right. This means maximizing your meals not eliminating them.

Excess calories are the biggest percentage of the problem pie chart, but the other pieces need to be identified so they can be recognized when looking to maximize your meals. In addition to chronic eating, there is the issue of food types that lead to inflammation that ultimately contributes to virtually every disease of the modern age. So, we don't need to count calories, we need to consider what those calories are made up of and how much inflammation is happening as a direct result from what's in our everyday recipes.

Acute inflammation is a response to injury that can feel like a burning in your muscles. It happens around an injury or a strain and it's a crucial part of the immune system response. Acute inflammation is characterized by the activation of white blood cells that rush to limit the damaged area to start the healing process.

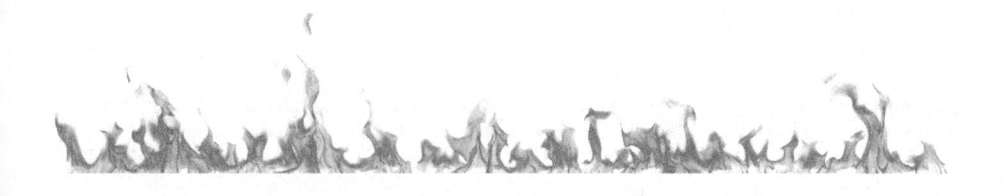

Presctiption Strength

Chronic inflammation is a whole different level of internal burning which is much more dangerous for your body. To put it simply, your immune system produces chemicals that cause inflammation. When those chemicals are limited to the site of an injury it's helpful and necessary. However, when they are produced in response to noninjuries, they are left free to rampage through your circulatory system causing all kinds of trouble in both the short term and long term.

Fire Starters

There are all kinds of noninjuries that can increase your level of inflammatory chemicals. These matches include:

1. Stress
2. Lack of Sleep
3. Excess Weight
4. Lack of adequate fiber
5. Certain foods

When you worry, your body is releasing chemicals. When you don't sleep, your body can compensate or activate certain chemicals. Your fat cells actually produce these proinflammatory chemicals as well. So do some foods or not having enough fiber.

Foods like sugars, simple starches and trans fats and saturated fats are all dangerous to some level. This is all very important when understanding how to design and maximize your meals. As you can imagine, the average meal in or out of your home consists of more than just high calories but dangerous types of calories that are likely to be very inflammatory.

#1 Killer in Men and Women

No where is inflammation more deadly than in your heart. This muscle the size of your fist receives oxygenated blood through tiny arteries called coronary arteries. When those arteries become clogged with fatty deposits and cholesterol, the blood flow to your heart is reduced. These fatty deposits are called plaque deposits. When a plaque deposit ruptures it can send pieces of plaque showering down your coronary arteries. Just like in your home plumbing, sooner or later one of these bigger pieces will get stuck and prohibit proper blood flow through an artery. Ultimately the result of these blocks will be a heart attack. In fact, the number one cause of death in men and women is heart disease.

Build Up and Breaks

Although we are still learning exactly how this process works, heart disease begins with chronic inflammation in the very delicate walls of your coronary arteries. We do know that the proinflammatory chemicals inure these sensitive walls which trigger your immune system to send white blood cells rushing to the area. The white blood cells combine with cells in your artery wall and form fatty streaks on the artery wall. Over time, lipids (fats) like cholesterol migrate to the site of the injury and the plaque starts to form and grow. Heart attacks commonly start when these plaques abruptly break apart.

The Scariest Part

The medically known process of atherosclerosis often has no symptoms. Cardiologists, like myself, measure a person's heart attack risk based on certain factors like your family history, whether or not you smoke, your weight and what you eat in your meals.

Presctiption Strength

For many people they will have no indication that a plaque is slowly moving through their coronaries like a time bomb. For tens of thousands of people every year, their first indication that they have serious heart disease is at the moment of a fatal heart attack. Although this is scary, my goal is not to strike fear in your heart but rather to educate you on where my motivation comes from when it comes to maximizing meals as well as the other pillars of perpetual health and wellbeing.

The Attraction of Easy Answers

Most doctors find themselves giving the same basic advice. Eat less, exercise more, get good sleep and reduce stress. Although all those things are true they aren't very helpful because it leaves to many unanswered questions. Unfortunately, the people wanting to answer these questions often offer magic bullets that don't work or don't work for most people or aren't sustainable. Still, people gravitate towards the easy and even though we can make complex things simple at SimpleMD®, there still needs to be a proven full proof plan that puts all the odds in your favor.

Pills and potions are everywhere to help you cleanse, detox, glow, shine, energize and more. Some work for some people. Some work some of the time and some work for a little while. I'm not going to spend too much time on this but when you maximize your meals, your need for pills and potions will greatly reduce.

Well Known Diets that Don't Always Work Well

Atkins Diet(s)

For many people, the word diet itself has become almost synonymous with the type of low-carb, high-protein eating regimen championed by Dr. Robert Atkins in his bestselling books *Dr. Atkins Diet Revolution* in 1972 and *Dr Atkins New Diet Revolution* in 1990. There are a few variations of this diet, including *The Zone, the South Beach Diet*, and even the *Keto Diet*, but they all operate on the same basic idea of lower carb and higher protein eating.

The problem? Not all carbs are created equal. Too much meat has it's own issues, and people don't always get enough exercise to take full advantage of this way of eating.

Paleo Diet(s)

Paleo diets are a more recent version of the traditional low-carb diet. The principle behind these diets is appealing and simple. According to their supporters, humans evolved millennia ago to eat and live a certain way. Back in ancient times, they say people were always on the move, getting near-constant exercise from walking and running. Their diet was comprised mostly of protein in the form of animal products, with some fat from organ meats mixed in with carbs being relatively rare because they had to be foraged. This program is designed to return people to their ancestral diet, but it also sounds like another repackaged low-carb diet.

Presctiption Strength

The problem? Not all carbs are created equal, too much meat has its own issues and people don't always get enough exercise to take full advantage of this way of eating.

Low Fat Diet(s)
Low fat eating plans were one of the original diet fads going back decades. They've mostly been replaced or gone out of style. Back when doctors were advising people to eat less fat to lose weight, it's fair to say we didn't really understand how dietary fats work. Like all carbs are not created equal, not all fats are created equal as well. Still, the concept looked good on paper and still has some merit when it comes to having less fat on your body, then maybe you should put less fat in it.

The problem? It would be best if you had certain kinds of fats for healthy living as well as weight loss. This will be discussed more when we share maximized meals.

Vegan Diet(s)
Vegan and vegetarian diets are constructed by avoiding or at least limiting all animal products from your diet. This isn't as much about losing weight for everyone who partakes in the program. Rather, it might also have to do with personal or spiritual beliefs. Like all diets that are successful, it's based on an idea that makes sense to some extent. In this case, there are health benefits to avoiding a lot of animal meats that may have been fed or drugged for the greatest growth potential.

The problem? It would be best if you had more protein and iron than you can typically get from a diet with no animal meat (including fish) of any kind. Protein has some amazing effects on our bodies when in moderation and in good quality.

So, what is the best way to eat (and maybe even live, for that matter)? Just what do our doctors at SimpleMD® prescribe? It is the Mediterranean Diet!

Maximize Your Meals with a Mediterranean Diet

Imagine a life where you wake up naturally with the sun and head to your kitchen for a cup of fresh coffee, perhaps with cream, to start your day. Afterwards, you walk or take a short bike ride to work in the morning hours and deal with your normal work issues. At lunch, you might return home for an hour or two to eat with your family or perhaps head to a local café with coworkers, where you enjoy a salad of fresh, local vegetables tossed with vinaigrette created from pure, first-pressed local olive oil. Perhaps you will have a piece of locally sourced fish as well.

When your workday ends around 5 p.m., you walk or bike home for a dinner that might include a small portion of locally raised meat, such as lamb, or perhaps more fish, and maybe some locally sourced goat cheese. And, of course, there are roasted vegetables tossed in more olive oil and another salad. You enjoy a glass of wine with dinner. Afterward, you have the evening to spend with your family or maybe taking a walk to the local plaza, then it's off to bed. Thus, we will reference the Mediterranean Diet as simply the Mediterranean Lifestyle, as both the process and the results are clearly more than just a particular combination of food ingredients.

Presctiption Strength

Ancient Wisdom

This forms the basis of what we now know as the "Mediterranean Lifestyle." It's really less of a diet and more of a pattern of life that operates by rhythms that are centuries old. The Mediterranean lifestyle focuses on plenty of exercise, lots of healthy fats from olive oil, and strong relationships. As doctors, we've known for more than a decade about the benefits of the Mediterranean Lifestyle. Less heart disease and cancer. Longer life. Less depression and mental health disorders. Improved quality of life in later years.

Whether reading or watching the news, the advice is constantly changing. One day, it reports avoiding eggs, then suddenly, eggs are fine again. Butter spent years on the naughty list while manufacturers rolled out tubs of colored and flavored trans fats that were supposed to be healthier, only to discover that those butter substitutes are a disaster.

**Check out our Mediterranean Recipes at SimpleMD.com*

The Right Way to do Research

Some of this confusion is related to legitimate issues with conducting nutrition research. In the world of medical research, the "gold standard" of studies is known as a double-blind, placebo-controlled study. In this kind of study, subjects are split into two groups. The first group is the control group, meaning they do not receive the medication or therapy but instead receive a sugar pill or fake therapy. The second group is the study group. Ideally, the study subjects have no idea which group they're in. This allows scientists to compare results from both groups and come up with objective, provable results.

In the world of nutrition, unfortunately, this type of study is virtually impossible. After all, who wants to be locked away in a lab somewhere for weeks or months while they are fed only certain foods? And even if you could find people willing to do this, most of the effects of diet are long-term and take years to measure.

This means that it's very hard actually to get good data on nutrition. Scientists
rely on a number of approaches, none of which are perfect. They use surveys (and we all know that people don't always tell the truth when they're asked about their diets!), and they use the kind of population studies I discussed in Chapter 1.

Ulterior Motives and Hidden Agendas
The second source of confusion over healthy nutrition has to do with profit motives. The sad fact is that there are a lot of snake-oil salespeople out there, pushing magical supplements or signing people up for expensive services that may or may not be based on sound science. The popularity of these shady products only proves my central point in writing this book: there is a huge thirst for good information that can help people lose weight and prevent chronic disease.

This is what led me to the Mediterranean Lifestyle in the first place. In a world of confusing or bad data, the benefits of this approach to eating and living are emerging as one of the few truly irrefutable truths. In this chapter, we're going to explore the building blocks of a healthy diet. Hopefully, by the end of this chapter, you'll have a basic understanding of what your body needs to thrive—and why our food culture can be so dangerous.

Demystifying Macronutrients

I want to start with a simple observation: the way you think about food and the way your body thinks about food might be dramatically different. To you, food might be about flavor, companionship, comfort, family, fun, and lots of other emotionally driven things. To your body, food is fuel and construction material.

We typically divide food into two large groups: macronutrients and micronutrients. If you think about food like your body does, macronutrients are the floor, walls, and ceiling of your building, while micronutrients are the fixtures, plumbing, and wiring. You need both but in different quantities.

When it comes to macronutrients, there are 3 types, and they form the foundation of every diet:

1. Carbohydrates. We talked a bit about carbohydrates in Chapter 1, but I want to dig a little deeper into what carbohydrates are exactly and how they fit into the Mediterranean lifestyle. An easy way to think of carbs is to think of them as energy. When you eat a carbohydrate, it is converted into glucose, which is the form of sugar that the body uses for energy. There are two kinds of carbs that fall into this category:

Simple Carbs, which include sugar, high fructose corn syrup, honey, and other carbohydrates. These are called 'simple' because they are easily broken down by the body and result in higher levels of blood sugar (glucose). In general, simple carbs are not a nutritious choice because they often have little nutrient value and result in a quick burst of energy followed by a crash. These types of carbs have also been implicated in America's ongoing obesity epidemic, especially the high fructose corn syrup found in so many soda drinks. Most nutrition experts advise people to stay away from any beverages containing high fructose corn syrup, and for good reason: these drinks are nothing but empty calories that wreak havoc with your metabolism and are directly related to weight gain. Any extra calories you consume as simple carbohydrates and that aren't needed for immediate energy are stored as fat.

Complex carbs which include carbs that form the foundation of the Mediterranean Lifestyle. The body also breaks down complex carbs into glucose, but because it is a more complex molecule, the breakdown takes much longer. Also, complex carbs are often packaged with yet another form of carbohydrate—fiber—that slows down the glucose absorption into your bloodstream even more. The result is lower "spikes" in your blood sugar levels, feeling fuller after a meal, and no post-carb crash. Examples of complex carbs include whole grains like oatmeal, vegetables, and most whole fruits. These complex carbohydrates form the basis of the Mediterranean Lifestyle, which is great news because they are also delicious!

2. <u>Fats</u>. Dietary fats are one of the most misunderstood of any macronutrient, thanks in part to misguided advice from nutrition experts and even government health agencies for years. Until relatively recently, all fats were lumped together into one big category, and people were told to avoid eating them. In truth, we now understand there are different kinds of fats, and some of them are absolutely essential to your health. Saturated Fats are the types of fats found in red meat and animal products, full-fat dairy, and some cooking oils. Saturated fats have

been linked to higher cholesterol, increased risk of heart disease, stroke, inflammation, and certain types of cancers. These fats should be eaten sparingly.

Trans fats are the real bad guys. Trans fats are not naturally occurring. Food producers invented them as a way to stabilize liquid vegetable oils through a process called hydrogenation (hence the term hydrogenated fat). These fats are very dangerous and have no health benefits. They have been linked to increased risk of heart attack, stroke, diabetes, atherosclerosis, and a host of other health issues. Because of recent changes in food labeling laws, food producers now have to list trans fats on the nutrition facts panel. Look for them and avoid them.

Unsaturated fats are the final type of fat, which is often called "good fat." Unsaturated fats include polyunsaturated and monounsaturated fats. This group includes the polyunsaturated fats omega-3 and omega-6 fatty acids, which can be found in cold-water fish. Monounsaturated fats are found in plant-based foods, including nuts and seeds, as well as olive oil. All of these fats are healthy and have been shown to protect your heart from heart disease, reduce inflammation, reduce the risk of certain cancers, and even reduce your risk of cognitive diseases like Alzheimer's disease. They are used throughout the body, including in the cell walls, and have been shown to help remove harmful cholesterol from your arteries.

The Mediterranean Lifestyle and lifestyle rely heavily on these fats, especially extra virgin olive oil. I'll talk more about this later on—especially the challenge of finding the real thing instead of buying adulterated fake olive oil from your corner grocery store—but the health benefits of consuming extra virgin olive oil are truly astounding. There are literally hundreds of high-quality scientific studies showing that this particular type of olive oil can suppress inflammation, help your heart, and even help control your weight. And the really good news? Authentic extra virgin olive oil is absolutely delicious.

*Check out our Mediterranean Recipes at SimpleMD.com

3. Protein. This is the third and final macronutrient, which has been enjoyed in a good run of great press for the last decade or so. Everyone from weight loss gurus to athletes have recommended dramatically increasing protein intake as a way to supercharge your metabolism. Protein is the building block used to create muscles and amino acids. It can be found in a variety of foods, including red meat, poultry, fish and seafood, and beans.

Protein itself is indeed a necessary part of any healthy diet, and according to the USDA, protein should be between 10 percent and 35 percent of an adult's daily calories. The problem arises in exactly how people are getting their protein. The American diet is heavily skewed toward consumption of red meat and dairy, perhaps best symbolized by that most American of foods: the cheeseburger. But dinner isn't the only time we're eating red meat. Sausages and bacon for breakfast. Lunch meats and cold cuts for lunch. And spaghetti meat sauce or chops for dinner.

Presctiption Strength

How Much is Too Much Meat?

When you consider that a single 8 oz. serving of beef could have 50 grams of protein—or about as much protein as anyone needs in a single day—you can see that we are gorging on protein. And unfortunately, most of these protein sources are also loaded with unhealthy fats, especially saturated fat, which is found in animal products. The Mediterranean Lifestyle also includes plenty of protein, but it comes from lean and clean sources, such as lean poultry and especially seafood. Fish, especially cold-water fish like salmon, is a great source of protein and healthy fats, including the critical omega-3 fatty acids.

By now, you're hopefully already seeing the outlines of the Mediterranean Lifestyle come into focus. It's heavy on whole fruits and healthy vegetables. It relies on healthy fats like extra virgin olive oil. And it focuses on lean and healthy proteins like poultry and seafood. If you're a cook, you can no doubt already see the delicious potential of eating like this! Trust me, when the people in the Mediterranean basin developed their cuisine centuries ago, they weren't thinking about heart disease or obesity. They were using fresh and local ingredients to create delicious foods—and that's exactly what the Mediterranean Lifestyle is all about.

Check out our Mediterranean Recipes at SimpleMD.com

No Chef Training Needed

And if you're not a cook, no worries. That's what SimpleMD® is all about: bringing the profound and proven benefits of the Mediterranean Lifestyle to everyone, no matter how busy you are. Our program has many simple suggestions that are helpful for everyone, no matter how busy you might be.

Demystifying Micronutrients

Aside from macronutrients, the other components of a healthy diet are micronutrients. Put simply, these are the vitamins and minerals. They are called micronutrients only because your body needs much smaller amounts of them to thrive in comparison to macronutrients.

Micronutrients are obtained through a healthy diet or, when necessary and recommended by your doctor, supplements.

Some of the major micronutrients include:
1. Iron
2. Calcium
3. Vitamins
4. Magnesium
5. Iodine
6. Zinc
7. Folate

*Maximize your meals right and you will get just about everything you need.

Deficiencies in any micronutrient can lead to adverse health consequences. For example, iron deficiency (anemia) is related to cognitive problems, while iodine deficiency can cause goiter development. Fortunately, true micronutrient deficiency in America is rare—no matter what the vitamin and supplement companies tell you.

Presctiption Strength

The Most Likely Problem is Too Much

Government agencies have launched ambitious programs to fortify table salt with iodine and flour with iron; both have been highly successful in reducing deficiencies in these two micronutrients. While there are areas of the world with widespread nutrient deficiencies, the issue in America is usually too much of a good thing, not too little. Too many calories. Too much sugar. Too much saturated fat. Too much salt.

So, if you want to take a multivitamin every day to ensure you're getting enough of the vitamins and minerals, talk to your doctor about it. Most doctors have no problem with daily multivitamins or supplementation with some of the other micronutrients and healthy fats (especially the omega-3 fatty acids). But really, the best way to ensure you're getting everything you need is by eating a varied and colorful diet of whole and wholesome foods—exactly the type of menu you'll find on the SimpleMD® Mediterranean Lifestyle.

The Way of Water

I mentioned this earlier, but I want to come back to this point because it's so important: drinking plenty of water is essential to this program, and it's especially important if you're on a GLP-1 medication.

GLP-1 medications are essentially hormones that help other molecules travel in and out of cells. This can lead to dehydration. It has also been our experience that many of the digestive side effects patients experience from the GLP-1 medications are improved significantly with extra water intake. Similarly, mild headaches, mild nausea, or even mild lightheadedness all completely abate with just a few extra glasses of water.

Many people ask whether water should be bubbly or flat, bottled or tap. We prefer flat water. Bubbles can give a temporary sensation of fullness due to the air taking up some more room in the stomach, but this quickly dissipates and might make people drink a bit less volume. Thus, we recommend flat water whenever possible.

When it comes to tap or bottled water, it's strictly a question of taste. Most water in the United States is safe to drink from the tap. It has been shown that slightly chilled water might have a very minor advantage to room temperature, but more studies need to be done to make this definitive.

Monitoring Your Urine

When it comes to how much, most people benefit from about six to eight glasses of water per day. Another way of monitoring your water intake is to try and keep your urine as clear as possible. This suggests excellent kidney filtration in most cases. The benefits of drinking plenty of water are many, and they include optimal weight loss and maintenance, so make sure you're very hydrated.

Research behind the Mediterranean Diet and Lifestyle

As a Cardiologist who has spent decades helping people prevent and treat heart disease, the Mediterranean Lifestyle has been on my radar for a long time—but when it came to sitting down to create SimpleMD®, there really was one moment that pushed me over the edge.

Presctiption Strength

It started in 2013, with the publication of the first results of a Spanish study known as the PREDIMED study, or Prevención con Dieta Mediterraneán study. This original study was published in the prestigious New England Journal of Medicine, and I want to share what really caught my attention.

Conducted by a researcher named Ramon Estruch and colleagues, the PREDIMED study looked at the dietary patterns of 7,447 people aged fifty-five to eighty years old. Almost 60 percent of them were women. The group was carefully selected for their lifestyle habits. Once in the study, they were divided into three study groups, given thorough health exams and histories, and then tracked for almost five years. Two of the three groups ate a recommended Mediterranean Lifestyle that included either a lot of extra virgin olive oil or mixed nuts. The third group was a control group that continued with their normal eating habits. There was no calorie restrictions in any diet group, and no requirement for additional exercise.

Oiling it Up

The initial results were striking. People in the study who ate extra nuts and extra virgin olive oil had a 30 percent reduction in the risk of a cardiovascular event (e.g., heart attack). Further, the extra virgin olive oil group experienced a significant reduction in the risk of stroke.

Fast forward a few years, as researchers continued to dig into the PREDIMED data, to an eye-catching study that was published in late 2015 on the benefits of the Mediterranean Lifestyle in regards to breast cancer.

Maximize Meals

As PREDIMED itself had shown, the Mediterranean Lifestyle could reduce the risk of heart disease and stroke. This wasn't too surprising; there was already plenty of data showing that the Mediterranean Lifestyle was good for your heart and arteries.

Reducing the Risk of Cancer

But now, a study came along that represented a paradigm shift in the way we think about nutrition and breast cancer. This new study, published in the Journal of the American Medical Association, looked at the rate of invasive breast cancer among women enrolled in the original PREDIMED study. And guess what? The study authors, led by Dr. Estefania Toledo, found that a diet high in extra virgin olive oil actually reduced the risk of breast cancer. This was the first randomized trial of any type showing that a particular diet could reduce the risk of breast cancer—and it all came down to extra virgin olive oil for the "primary prevention of breast cancer."

This is deeply exciting because it shows that the Mediterranean Lifestyle isn't a one-trick diet. It's not "only" good for heart disease. In fact, the Mediterranean Lifestyle is about growing good health in every area of life.

Mediterranean Style Food Pyramid

Most of us are familiar with the government food pyramid, with its comfortingly familiar stacks of suggested food groups. When it was first introduced, the bottom layer of the food pyramid was built solely on grains (carbs), with the next layer up comprising fruits and vegetables. After we learned more about the dangers of bingeing on carbs, it was revised in 2005 and reintroduced as MyPyramid. This version was much less intuitive and featured colored wedges running up the side of the pyramid.

Presciption Strength

In 2011, only six years after MyPyramid was introduced, the government rolled out MyPlate, this time showing a plate divided into quadrants based on recommended food servings, with a separate glass for the dairy group. In this version, fruits and vegetables make up half of the plate, with the rest divided between grains and protein (e.g., meat and beans).

According to the government guidelines under MyPlate, a healthy diet would comprise:
- Vegetables: 40 percent
- Fruit: 10 percent
- Grains: 30 percent
- Protein: 20 percent
- Dairy: Unspecified, but daily

Don't Forget the Fat

This version was considered an improvement, but it still left a lot to be desired when it comes to following the scientifically validated principles of the Mediterranean Lifestyle. For example, the government food plate makes no effort to distinguish between healthy fats and unhealthy fats. Likewise, there's little science backing up the idea that adults should be consuming any amount of dairy on a daily basis. Likewise, it only makes the most vague recommendations on the type of grains people should eat.

But I'm not here to critique the government's recommendations. Instead, I want to introduce you to a simple new food pyramid based on the Mediterranean Lifestyle. This "new" food pyramid is actually more than a decade old, but it's still new to many people.

Maximize Meals

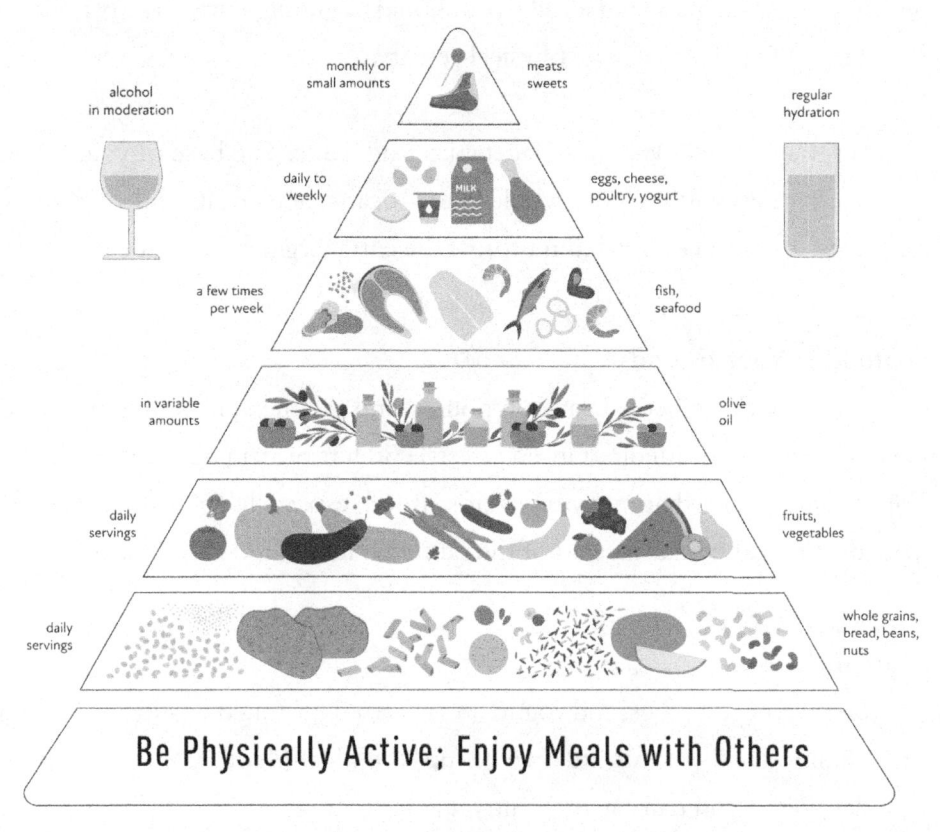

The Mediterranean Diet Food Pyramid

- alcohol in moderation
- monthly or small amounts — meats, sweets
- regular hydration
- daily to weekly — eggs, cheese, poultry, yogurt
- a few times per week — fish, seafood
- in variable amounts — olive oil
- daily servings — fruits, vegetables
- daily servings — whole grains, bread, beans, nuts

Be Physically Active; Enjoy Meals with Others

Let's take a look at some of the prominent features of this modified pyramid and how it fits into the Mediterranean Lifestyle and the SimpleMD® program.

Moderate exercise is an everyday thing! But before you think, "Oh great, another doctor telling me I need to spend more time in the gym," think about the actual types of exercise that long-lived people in the Mediterranean basin

Presctiption Strength

get. They walk a lot. They play outdoor sports. They dance. All of this counts as healthy physical activity, and ideally, you should be getting thirty to sixty minutes every day of light to moderate physical activity.

It is built on whole grains, vegetables, and fruits. The base of your diet is varied and healthy. It includes whole grains, beans, nuts, fruits and vegetables, herbs, and even spices. And don't forget the extra virgin olive oil, or EVOO!

Seafood is Your Friend

The American diet is heavy on poultry and red meat, including pork and beef. In contrast, the Mediterranean Lifestyle prefers protein from the sea. Why? For the simple fact that many types of seafood, especially cold-water fish, are loaded with healthy fats instead of the saturated fats found in red meat.

More or Less

Poultry, cheese, eggs, and yogurt are preferred in limited quantities. Instead of breaking dairy out into its own group, the ideal Mediterranean Lifestyle includes yogurt and dairy with poultry and eggs. If you have a real craving for dairy, I'd always recommend going with a low-fat or reduced-fat yogurt instead of cheese or whole-fat milk products. Yogurt is loaded with healthy bacteria that help keep your digestion moving and power your immune system. Eggs are also okay, especially as newer research is showing that the concern over cholesterol in eggs is overstated but try to limit your consumption to three or four eggs a week.

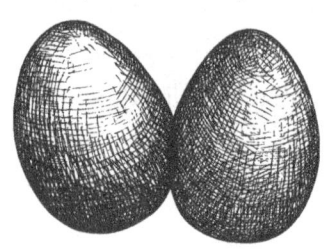

Meat and sweets should be eaten sparingly. What does this mean? I'd suggest aiming to eat red meat once a week and switch out your dessert of ice cream with fresh fruit. Water and wine both make the list. Water is essential for life and good health, so you should be drinking plenty of water every day.

As for wine, red wine contains a very powerful ingredient that has significant health benefits—but this must be balanced against the dangers of consuming alcohol. Recent research has suggested that no amount of alcohol consumption is truly safe. When you drink alcohol, it must be detoxified in the liver, which can take a serious toll over time. Excessive drinking is one of the leading causes of cirrhosis of the liver, an incurable, progressive, and frequently fatal liver disease. Excessive alcohol consumption is also known to impair judgment, reduce inhibitions, contribute to depression and other mood disorders, and cause damage to unborn children, and it is listed as a contributing factor in drunk driving accidents and domestic violence cases every day.

Check out our Mediterranean Recipes at SimpleMD.com
(All of these are examples of Maximizing Your Mealtime!)

With this in mind, instead of adding alcohol to your diet, I suggest focusing on the substances in red wine that offer health benefits. Perhaps this is not surprising, but what makes red wine so powerful begins with the grapes. Wine grapes are full of powerful antioxidants called polyphenols. According to the American Journal of Clinical Nutrition, polyphenols are a particular type of antioxidant that is best known for preventing diseases like heart disease and cancer. They are commonly found in medicinal plants and are known to take an active role in enzyme activity and cell health. It's also fair to say that research into polyphenols is still relatively new—this branch of science didn't really open up until the last fifteen years or so, with an explosion of research into the varied benefits of polyphenols. Polyphenols can be found in green tea, coffee, herbs and spices, fruits, vegetables… and red grapes.

Wines Secret Health Ingredient

The chief polyphenol in red wine is called resveratrol. Resveratrol was discovered early in the twentieth century by a Japanese researcher, but it wasn't until a Harvard scientist published positive findings in the prestigious journal Nature in 2003 that global research on resveratrol really took off. Today, many of the major health benefits of red wine are credited directly to its high resveratrol concentration, and there are almost eight thousand studies on resveratrol alone in the National Institutes of Health database. Resveratrol has even attracted attention from life extension researchers, who believe that it may be able to extend cell life and someday be used to prolong human life. While researchers are still digging to uncover exactly how resveratrol benefits human health, there is plenty we do know. Here is just a sampling of its proven benefits:

Good for the Heart

It helps protect the heart against ischemic heart disease. This is the most common type of heart disease and the cause of most heart attacks. While resveratrol does have significant benefits, considering the emerging data on the health risks of alcohol consumption, I'm not recommending adding red wine or any alcohol to your diet. If you already have an occasional drink as part of your lifestyle, my advice is to make it red wine. Ultimately, though, the health benefits of abstaining outweigh any perceived benefits of drinking, so if you are interested in the benefits of resveratrol, you can focus on supplements or obtain it through the SimpleMD™ protein bars. As always, if you are considering using alcohol as part of your diet, talk it over with your doctor.

Fighting Cancer, Alzheimer's, and Dementia

Resveratrol, along with other plant chemicals, is known to target and disrupt the creation of cancer cells. Alzheimer's disease is one of the most pressing health issues facing our aging population. It is the primary cause of dementia and one of the leading causes of death in the United States. Exciting new research is showing that resveratrol can be an important part of a multi-faceted approach to treating and slowing the progression of Alzheimer's.

Resveratrol has been shown to modify certain brain chemicals that are closely linked to increased risk of obesity, diabetes, and metabolic syndrome, which are all closely related to increased risk of heart disease as well as a constellation of other health issues.

Even depression, autism and bipolar disorder

Through its ability to support healthy brain function and regular neurochemicals, resveratrol can help prevent depression and bipolar disorder and, in some smaller studies, has been shown to reduce the risk of autism.

With all of these benefits, I'm recommending that you consider incorporating a bit of red wine consumption into your diet if it fits your lifestyle. That said, if you abstain or don't want to take on the other risks associated with drinking alcohol, the good news is we've incorporated high-quality red wine into the SimpleMD® bars so that you may get some of the benefits without the downsides of excessive alcohol. Others have suggested capsule-based supplementation to be beneficial as well. I would recommend that you discuss these options with your clinician.

Presctiption Strength

There is a very good reason extra virgin olive oil (EVOO) is included in the very base of the Mediterranean Lifestyle food pyramid. Put simply, it's an incredibly healthy fat that you should be consuming every day. EVOO is loaded with healthy monounsaturated fats and powerful antioxidants. In this chapter, we're going to take a look at what makes this oil so powerful—and the steps you need to take to ensure you're getting its full benefit.

Highly Processed is a Problem

EVOO is one of the purest and simplest cooking oils in existence. Without going into great detail, most of the vegetable oils in your local supermarket are highly processed and purified. They are built to last for a long time in your cupboard without oxidizing and without changing their taste. To accomplish this, the oils are often extracted from their source (like soybeans or seeds) with solvents, then pasteurized at high temperatures, and treated with a procession of chemicals that might include phosphoric acid, sodium hydroxide, aldehydes, and others to achieve a bland, colorless, long-lasting product.

EVOO, on the other hand, is created from the first press of freshly harvested olives. Once the olives are pressed, the resulting juice is strained, bottled, and shipped.

A good bottle of EVOO should actually taste like the olives it came from, and it should be fresh. In many ways, this product is much closer to wine than to other cooking oils. Depending on where it's from and its quality, EVOO can be fruity, buttery and smooth, spicy, peppery, or just slightly bitter. In Italy, there's an entire profession devoted to tasting and rating EVOO for purity and flavor.

As you might imagine, this product is hard to produce—but the benefits are profound. In addition to the shocking study that I cited earlier, which shows that EVOO can actually reduce the risk of invasive breast cancer. Consider these findings:

Extra virgin olive oil has been shown to protect the inner lining of coronary arteries and help lower blood pressure in women diagnosed with high blood pressure.

A review of all the published benefits of EVOO found that it helped reduce inflammation in the coronary arteries, may help lower total cholesterol, reduce the formation of blood clots, and provide additional evidence that it supports healthy arteries. EVOO has been shown to help prevent strokes in the elderly.

Check out our Mediterranean Recipes at SimpleMD.com

Did You Know?
The Mediterranean Lifestyle is the only diet scientifically proven to improve bone health and reduce the risk of hip fractures, according to the Journal of the American Medical Association in March 2016.

In lab studies, EVOO has been shown to slow tumor growth in colon cancer. Consumption of olive oil appears to support healthy brain function and might even protect against depression. It has even been shown to benefit skin health. Leading dermatologists like Dr. Glynis Ablon, a professor at UCLA and a frequent expert on the TV show The Doctors, have long recommended the Mediterranean Lifestyle for healthy skin, in part because of the EVOO. Similarly, Dr. Leslie Baumann, New York Times best-selling author of The Skin Type Solution, writes that "your skin might just thank you" for consuming enough EVOO. She writes, "A report I authored in 2007 that was published in the Journal of Pathology discusses the role of antioxidants like vitamin E in contributing to radiant, younger-looking skin. The healthy amount of vitamin E found in olive oil has been shown to be successful in neutralizing free radicals and photoaging from UVA rays that damage skin cells, helping to maintain the appearance of youth.

Look Younger?

In addition, olive oil contains linoleic acid, a component of skin that helps prevent water from evaporating (water is another substance that promotes a youthful appearance). People who are deficient in linoleic acid can develop dry, flaky skin. Since linoleic acid is not produced naturally in the body, it needs to be supplemented in the diet or topically applied to the skin."

In fact, there is a convincing body of research showing that olive oil can be used as a lip moisturizer, after-sun treatment, deep hair conditioner, and bath oil, and may even help prevent acne thanks to its high content of omega-3 fatty acids.

I could go on—there are almost eight hundred peer-reviewed studies on EVOO in the National Institutes of Health database—but you get the point. EVOO is unique among cooking oils for its ability to support a healthy heart, brain, and vascular system, and newer research is even suggesting it reduces the risk of certain types of cancer.

So, does that mean you should run out right now and buy the first bottle of EVOO you see on the supermarket shelves? Not exactly. Unfortunately, when it comes to EVOO, what you see isn't always what you get.

Watch out for Fake EVOO

In early 2016, the respected news magazine 60 Minutes ran a shocking story on Italian extra virgin olive oil. According to 60 Minutes, the Italian olive oil industry has been thoroughly infiltrated by the Mafia. Yes, you read that right. Just like in the movie The Godfather, where the Corleone family was heavily involved in exporting olive oil, real-life Mafia figures have corrupted the Italian olive oil business. How exactly? By selling fake products.

According to 60 Minutes, an astonishing 75 to 80 percent of Italian EVOO sold in the United States has been adulterated, diluted, or mislabeled and does not meet the legal definition for EVOO. The most common form of fraud? Taking a standard oil, like sunflower oil, and adding chlorophyll and beta-carotene to make it look and smell somewhat like the real thing, while in fact, the bottle contains little to no EVOO at all!

Check out our Mediterranean Recipes at SimpleMD.com

I was shocked when I saw this report. It's bad enough to defraud consumers by selling them a fake product, but when that product is also linked directly to better health, it takes on a new dimension.

First, I would stress that there is a difference between other cooking oils, regular olive oil, and extra virgin olive oil. Only a true EVOO is loaded with

Presctiption Strength

the ideal mix of antioxidants. Only a true EVOO provides the purest and best source of monounsaturated fatty acids. The fact is that there is no substitute for the real thing, both in terms of taste and health benefits.

How Many Table Spoons of EVOO?

Once we agree that almost everyone should be consuming EVOO, the next question is: how much? A traditional Mediterranean-style diet calls for eating about eight to ten olives or ingesting three to four tablespoons of olive oil every day. The Food and Drug Administration recommends about two tablespoons daily. The PREDIMED study, the largest and most definitive scientific study on the benefits of olive oil, used four tablespoons a day as its benchmark. Because of the outstanding results in the PREDIMED study, I recommend four tablespoons every day.

Fortunately, extra virgin olive oil is so delicious that it's not hard to get those few tablespoons every day. You can use olive oil as a dipping sauce for fresh bread or in salad dressings for example.

*Check out our Mediterranean Recipes at SimpleMD.com

Where to Look in the Store

If you're at a grocery store, however, look for varieties that are cold pressed and organic, and specifically seek out those that are certified by the International Olive Oil Association or the California Olive Oil Council. High-quality extra virgin olive oil possesses a pleasant aroma, a deep green hue, and a delicious taste, often with a hint of peppery bitterness.

Maximize Meals

If you haven't realized it yet, Extra Virgin Olive Oil is a big part of a Maximized Mealtime!

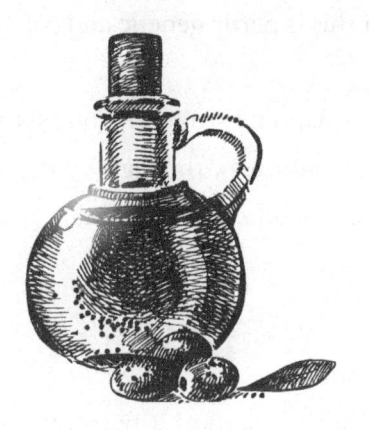

The Truth about Fasting

Some form of fasting has been popular for weight loss for many years now, often with disappointing results. Among my patients, I've seen people try to fast up to twenty hours a day or fast completely for a day or two. Unfortunately, the results of these ad-hoc approaches haven't been great. In many cases, people lose weight at first but then gain it back as soon as they go back on a "regular" eating schedule.

The Achievable Sustainable Approach

The good news is there is a reasonable and achievable approach to intermittent fasting that we have shown great success in our practices with. Following these steps blunts the inevitable hunger that derails most people. Not surprisingly, fasting causes a surge in hormones that cause food cravings as your body attempts to prepare itself against famine. These cravings can be almost impossible to overcome. Remember that your body has a set point when

Presctiption Strength

it comes to weight. A caloric deficit in the form of fasting will set off internal alarm bells that your natural set point is threatened and it's time to load up on calories. Studies suggest this is partly genetic and partly environmental.

As I mentioned in Chapter 1, though, your set point isn't your destiny. Studies show that if you can break through your set point, it is possible to reorient your metabolism around a new set point in as little as ten weeks, leading to permanent weight loss.

Accelerate Your Metabolism

Maximized Mealtime™ is a good way to reset your metabolism, and it has other benefits as well. David Sinclair's work from Harvard, as well as many others, has shown that the human body seems to prefer occasional reductions in calories. During even minor periods of fasting, the body responds by improving cellular protective mechanisms, including anti-inflammatory and anti-destructive pathways that may positively affect longevity and aging, as well as contributing to weight loss.

Our method is designed to help you reduce your calorie intake as much as possible without discomfort. If people don't feel as comfortable, it is much more likely the strategy will fail. Our SimpleMD® plan allows patients to enjoy the long-term benefits of eating less.

8 On, 16 Off

If even partial fasting sounds challenging, don't worry! Our 8-hour unrestricted eating window, followed by the 16-hour food break (8 hours of which is sleeping), will surprise most people with its ease. The program is easiest to start while on a GLP-1 medication. However, even off the medications, avoiding calories in the early morning and evening can quickly become a positive habit.

We understand this approach can seem overwhelming at first, but the SimpleMD® program is designed to help you be successful. In addition to the GLP-1s, our SimpleMD® protein bars are a great way to supplement your diet and stick to your eating plan. SimpleMD® protein bars have been routinely used for many years as an easy solution when traditional Mediterranean Lifestyle food preparation is inconvenient or unavailable. These bars have been carefully designed to provide a healthy, low-calorie boost while also giving you two of the greatest benefits of the Mediterranean Diet: olive oil and the resveratrol found in red wine. This book is not intended to be a sales tool for the bars. However, through the years, so many have enjoyed them and they seem to be a good "life hack" when one doesn't have the time to find an optimal food choice. There are other applicable protein bars and meal replacements on the market, and we are in the process of properly reviewing them and will add them to our website (along with easy to make recipes) to ensure variety and options for all.

Presctiption Strength

More Control, Less Cravings

Certain protein bars have been shown to have a number of health benefits, including: Hunger Control—Protein has been shown to increase feelings of fullness and decrease hunger, making it an effective tool for weight management. Lower calorie protein bars are a convenient way to increase protein intake and control hunger between meals.

Not Just for Weightlifters

Muscle Building and Repair—Protein is an essential nutrient for building and repairing muscle, and it's essential for maintaining a healthy metabolism. By increasing protein intake through lower calorie protein bars, individuals can improve muscle mass and enhance their overall metabolism, helping to achieve and maintain a healthy weight.

Reduced Caloric Intake—By choosing lower calorie protein bars as a snack option, individuals can reduce their overall caloric intake. Additionally, the protein content in these bars can help to reduce cravings for high calorie, sugary snacks.

Can certain types of eating mimic fasting?

The short answer is YES. Dr. Valter Longo from the University of Southern California is involved in Nobel Prize-winning research on this very idea.

He and his colleagues at L-Nutra and Prolon have developed some well-designed nutritional products designed to essentially "trick" the body into gaining many of the benefits of fasting with less….fasting!

MAXIMIZED MEAL TIME

We recommend splitting your day into twelve hours of fasting, which includes sleep; and twelve hours of Maximized Meal Time (MMT).

The first and last two hours of your MMT can be augmented by eating a 130-calorie SimpleMD protein bar. High in fiber and protein, they are the perfect snack to help you stay in a "fasting state" in the morning or start one in the evening.

Limiting the time you eat doesn't mean limiting your choices. Choose sensible foods and snacks and get plenty of sleep. Here's what a typical day should look like:

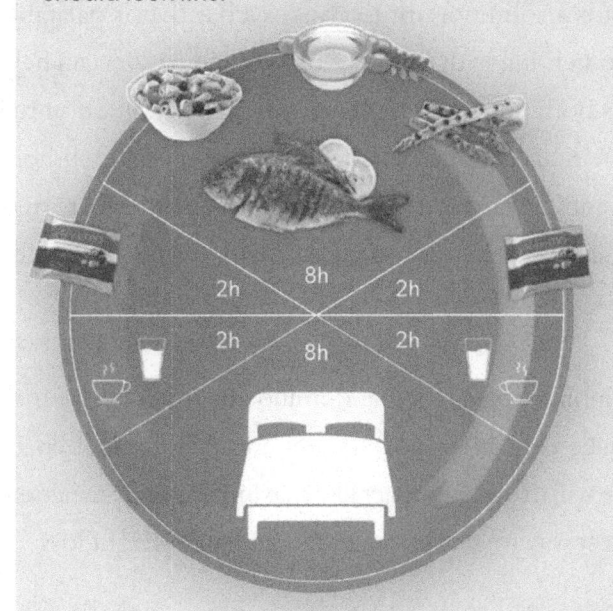

Enjoy traditional Mediterranean Diet foods such as lean protein from fish or chicken, vegetables, and extra virgin olive oil.

We recommend at least 8 hours of sleep each night. And do not eat at least two hours before you go to bed and for the first two hours after you wake up. Enjoy coffee or tea, but skip the added sugar!

SimpleMD®

Presctiption Strength

How to Buy the Perfect Bar

If you prefer not to use SimpleMD® bars, there are plenty of other options. When you're shopping for healthy protein bars, here are a few things to take into consideration:

Nutritional Content—It is important to choose lower calorie protein bars that are high in protein (8–10 grams) and low in added sugars. Additionally, bars should contain healthy ingredients, such as nuts, seeds, and added fiber, to maximize their nutritional benefits.

Taste—While it is important to choose a lower calorie protein bar with good nutritional content, it is also important to choose a bar that is palatable and enjoyable to eat. Experimenting with different brands and flavors can help individuals find a bar that is both nutritious and satisfying. The addition of red wine into SimpleMD® protein bars has had a beneficial effect on taste, without appreciable alcohol, while adding the benefits of resveratrol. Other bars may have other benefits, but be sure your calories and ingredients are in line with the principles outlined above.

As I stated at the beginning, this is the big domino and a relatively small thing you can do that will make a big difference. No amount of exercise, sleep, or anything else for that matter will make an impact like maximizing your mealtime will. Eating right is the fastest way to get the biggest sustainable weight loss.

As a matter of fact, the more you eat "right" the more you can do some of the other things "wrong" or not at all. That's how powerful this part is.

Maximize Meals

Thus, a crucial part of the SimpleMD® full medical weight loss program has lots of tips on easy recipes, meals, and food resources. It can be quite confusing and challenging to get all the right ingredients and meals together, so we offer easy options so people can make the first successful step in their journey.

Here are some example meals that we can provide the complete recipe for:

Baked Falafel: Mix chickpeas, onion, garlic, parsley, cumin, salt, and pepper. Shape into balls and bake until crispy. Serve with tahini sauce.

Stuffed Grape Leaves: Roll grape leaves filled with rice, lemon juice, dill, and mint. Bake or boil until tender.

Hummus with Vegetables: Blend chickpeas, tahini, lemon juice, and garlic. Serve with sliced cucumbers, carrots, and bell peppers.

Grilled Eggplant Rolls: Slice eggplant and grill. Fill with ricotta cheese, sun-dried tomatoes, and basil.

Roasted Chickpeas: Toss chickpeas with olive oil, cumin, paprika, and salt. Roast in the oven until crispy.

Tzatziki with Pita Chips: Mix Greek yogurt, cucumber, garlic, dill, lemon juice, and salt. Serve with pita chips.

**Check out our Mediterranean Recipes at SimpleMD.com*

YOU DON'T HAVE TO HAVE IT ALL FIGURED OUT TO MOVE FORWARD

CHAPTER 6
Mindful Movements

The modern world no longer moves, which has become a contributing factor to an increase in obesity and its related health issues. One of the most common features of today's health tech, like a Fitbit watch, is to remind us to move. SimpleMD®'s philosophy believes in the power of movement for both physical and mental well-being.

Through our experience, research, and evaluation of numerous studies, we have summarized two primary types of basic exercise that can help individuals achieve a healthy weight loss: mindful aerobic and resistance activities, or what we like to characterize as Meaningful Movement.

This chapter is all about the importance of exercises, as well as providing examples of these movements, and to present some evidence to support their effectiveness in promoting weight loss and overall health.

Kickstart Your Cardio

Aerobic exercise, also known as cardiovascular exercise, is a type of physical activity that involves repetitive movements of large muscle groups, such as walking, jogging, swimming, or cycling. These activities have been proven to be effective in promoting weight loss and providing general health benefits.

Brisk walking, for example, is a highly accessible and efficient aerobic exercise.

Presctiption Strength

Research has demonstrated that brisk walking can lead to significant weight loss and health improvements. A recent study showed that individuals who engaged in a brisk walking program for 12 weeks experienced a significant reduction in body fat and an increase in aerobic fitness.

Increasing Your Heart Rate, Decreasing Diseases

Additionally, brisk walking has been associated with a decreased risk of chronic diseases, such as cardiovascular disease and type 2 diabetes. There is so much published data on this form of exercise that an exhaustive summary is beyond the scope of this chapter. However, we wanted to point out a few simple examples that illustrate the benefits of aerobic activities in achieving optimal healthful weight loss results.

Use Your Muscles

Resistance training, also known as strength training or weightlifting, is a type of exercise that involves working against a force to build muscle strength and endurance. Examples of resistance activities include push-ups, squats, and lunges.

Resistance training can have a significant impact on weight loss efforts and overall health. Studies have shown that resistance training can lead to an increase in lean muscle mass, which helps boost metabolism, enabling the body to burn more calories at rest. This can contribute to sustained weight loss and improved body composition. Furthermore, resistance training has been shown to enhance bone density, decrease the risk of injury, and improve balance and coordination.

Your Heart is a Muscle

In addition to these benefits, resistance training can also improve cardiovascular health. A study by Strasser et al. (2010) found that resistance training led to significant improvements in cardiovascular risk factors, such as reduced blood pressure and improvements in lipid profiles. This suggests that resistance training alone can play an essential role in weight loss and overall health.

Again, there is much published on the benefits of various types of resistance training. Suffice it to say for the purpose of this introductory chapter, adding resistance training to one's weight loss journey can only benefit the healthful weight loss results.

Combine Activities to Multiply Results

While both aerobic and resistance exercises offer numerous health benefits, combining these two types of activities can lead to even greater results. A meta-analysis showed that the combination of aerobic and resistance training resulted in increased weight loss and improved body composition compared to aerobic exercise alone. Additionally, engaging in both types of exercise improved cardiovascular health, muscular strength and overall function. There is also proof that muscle helps burn fat, so increasing muscle is also reducing fat when done right.

For individuals seeking medium to low-impact exercises that still provide high calorie burning, there are several effective options to consider.

Presctiption Strength

Here are the Top 5 Most Efficient Exercises:

1. <u>Cycling</u>: Cycling is an excellent low-impact exercise that can be done outdoors or on a stationary bike. It engages the large muscles of your legs, leading to significant calorie burning. You can control the intensity, making it suitable for people of different fitness levels. Additionally, cycling is a fun and enjoyable activity that can be done alone or with friends.

2. <u>Swimming</u>: Swimming is a full-body workout that puts minimal stress on the joints. It is an ideal choice for individuals with joint issues or those who are overweight. Swimming can burn a substantial number of calories as it works various muscle groups simultaneously. Moreover, the water's buoyancy provides a soothing effect on the body.

3. <u>Rowing</u>: Rowing is an underrated yet highly effective exercise for calorie burning. Whether using a rowing machine or rowing on the water, this exercise engages your upper body, core, and legs. It can burn a high number of calories while promoting cardiovascular health. Proper rowing technique is essential to prevent injury and maximize calorie burning.

4. <u>Elliptical Training</u>: The elliptical machine is a low-impact option that mimics movements similar to running without the high impact on joints. This exercise targets both the upper and lower body, making it an efficient calorie-burning workout. Most elliptical machines allow you to adjust the resistance and incline to intensify your workout.

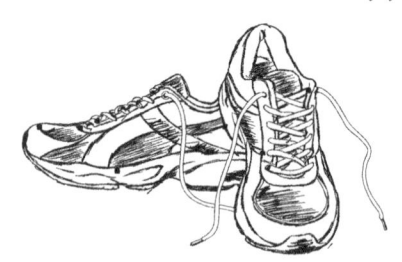

5. <u>Power Walking</u>: Power walking, also known as brisk walking, is an accessible and effective exercise for calorie burning. Walking at a faster pace can significantly increase your heart rate and engage multiple muscle groups. While it may be lower impact than running, it can still burn a substantial number of calories, especially when done consistently for longer durations.

Remember that the number of calories burned during these exercises will vary depending on factors such as body weight, intensity, and duration of the workout. It's also essential to combine these exercises with a balanced diet to achieve optimal results in weight management and overall health.

Before starting any exercise program, especially if you have any underlying health conditions or concerns, it's advisable to consult with a healthcare professional or fitness expert to ensure the chosen exercises are safe and suitable for your individual needs.

Not a lot of Time?

When it comes to efficient full-body workouts that engage multiple muscle groups in a short amount of time, compound exercises are the way to go. Compound exercises involve movement at more than one joint and engage numerous muscles simultaneously. They are highly effective for building strength, increasing muscle mass, and burning calories efficiently. Both men and women can benefit from compound exercises, as they provide comprehensive workouts that target various muscle groups.

Presctiption Strength

Here are some of the Best Compound Exercises:

1. <u>Squats:</u> Squats are a powerhouse exercise that primarily targets the muscles of the lower body, including quadriceps, hamstrings, and glutes. They also engage the core for stability. Squats are beneficial for both men and women, helping to build strong legs and improve overall lower body strength.

2. <u>Deadlifts</u>: Deadlifts work the muscles of the back, including the erector spinae and lats, as well as the glutes and hamstrings. They also engage the core muscles for stabilization. Deadlifts are excellent for developing a strong posterior chain (the muscles on the backside of your body) and can benefit both men and women.

3. <u>Bench Press</u>: Bench presses target the chest, shoulders, and triceps. While often associated with upper body strength, they can be effective for both men and women. Women, in particular, can benefit from bench presses to enhance upper body strength and muscle tone.

4. <u>Pull-Ups/Chin-Ups</u>: Pull-ups and chin-ups are fantastic compound exercises that engage the muscles of the back, particularly the latissimus dorsi, along with the biceps and shoulders. While pull-ups might be more challenging for some women initially due to differences in upper body strength, with consistent training, they can be a valuable addition to a workout routine for both genders.

5. <u>Overhead Press</u>: The overhead press targets the shoulders, triceps, and upper back muscles. It's a great exercise for developing strong and well-rounded shoulders. Women can benefit from overhead presses to enhance shoulder strength and stability.

6. <u>Lunges</u>: Lunges are excellent for working the lower body muscles, including quadriceps, hamstrings, and glutes. They also engage the core for balance. Lunges can be beneficial for both men and women to improve leg strength and stability.

7. <u>Rows</u>: Rowing exercises, whether with a barbell, dumbbells, or a rowing machine, target the back muscles, biceps, and rear deltoids. Rows help balance out the muscles worked during pressing exercises and are valuable for overall upper body strength and posture.

It's important to note that there's no strict division between exercises that are better for men versus women. Both genders can benefit from a variety of compound exercises to promote strength, muscle development, and overall fitness. The choice of exercises may depend on individual goals, fitness levels, and any specific considerations. It's always recommended to consult with a fitness professional or personal trainer to tailor an exercise program to your unique needs and preferences.

Personalizing Your Physical Training

It is crucial to recognize that every individual has unique needs, preferences, and limitations when it comes to exercise. Factors such as age, fitness level, and personal goals should be considered when designing an exercise program. By tailoring the type and intensity of exercise to each person, it is possible to maximize the benefits of physical activity while minimizing the risk of injury. Some patients have the luxury of abundant internal motivation, others hire personal trainers to assist their journeys.

Presctiption Strength

Coaches and Trainers

SimpleMD® has developed a basic system of coaching that helps motivate and sustain many of our patients in their healthful weight loss journey. To stay motivated and committed to a regular exercise routine, many individuals can benefit from working with a coaching system. A coaching system provides support, guidance, and accountability, helping individuals stay on track and achieve their fitness goals. It has been found that coaches can also help individuals identify the most suitable exercises, monitor progress, and motivate, ensuring that the benefits of a consistent exercise routine continue to progress.

Adding Mindfulness to the Mix

Mindful exercise means being present and focused during workouts, which can lead to numerous physical and mental health benefits. By concentrating on the task at hand, you can enhance your performance, reduce stress, and gain a greater sense of satisfaction from exercise.

Benefits of mindful exercise include improved mental health, such as reduced stress, depression, and anxiety, as well as better sleep. Physical health improvements can also be observed, such as increased cardiovascular health, lower BMI, and fasting glucose levels. Mindful exercise also helps strengthen your commitment to your workout routine, leading to higher levels of satisfaction.

Mindful Fitness Strategies

Set a purpose for each workout, focusing on something specific, like strengthening particular muscles or challenging yourself. Please pay attention to your body, noticing how it feels during the exercise and avoiding comparisons to others.

Remember why you're exercising and the benefits it brings.

- Slow down and focus on each movement, especially during strength training exercises.
- Remind yourself to breathe, using it as an "attention anchor" to stay present.
- End on a positive note, giving yourself time to cool down, stretch, and appreciate the workout's effects.

By incorporating mindful exercise into your routine, you can achieve greater physical and mental well-being and, ultimately, a healthier lifestyle.

In conclusion, Meaningful Movement, SimpleMD®'s approach to basic exercise, emphasizes the importance of incorporating both mindful aerobic and resistance activities into a regular exercise routine. Brisk walking and push-ups are just two examples of exercises that can be easily incorporated into daily life, leading to significant weight loss and improved general health when combined with our other methods. By tailoring exercise programs to individual needs and working with a coaching system for motivation (like our dietary coaching), our experience suggests that this is the best final ingredient to an overall recipe for healthy weight loss and long-term.

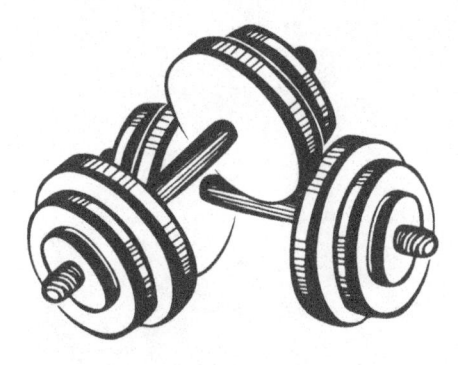

PART 3
Results

TO PROTECT YOUR ENERGY...

It's okay to not answer a call.
It's okay to change your mind.
It's okay to want to be alone.
It's okay to take a day off.
It's okay to do nothing.
It's okay to speak up.
It's okay to let go.

CHAPTER 7
More Rest

You need to not just sleep but enter various stages of sleep regularly even nightly. There is Light sleep that makes up most of your night REM sleep that makes up probably the second biggest amount of sleep you have a night and then you have Deep sleep. These different sleep cycles and states of rest are almost always necessary to reach your peak performance throughout any day.

Good sleep lengthens your fuse, giving you more patience, helps you focus, make better decisions and even speeds up your reaction time or alertness in any situation. The sleep industry is a billion-dollar industry and in some ways is almost as big as the weight loss industry. In fact, they really go hand in hand. It's definitely a part of the 8 Pillars of Perpetual Health and Well Being. Bottom line, you need more rest especially when you are eating right, exercising more regularly putting the 8 pillars to work in your life.

The type of rest required can vary based on different situations, such as after exercise, when you're sick, or following a stressful period. Rest is essential for recovery, healing, and overall well-being.

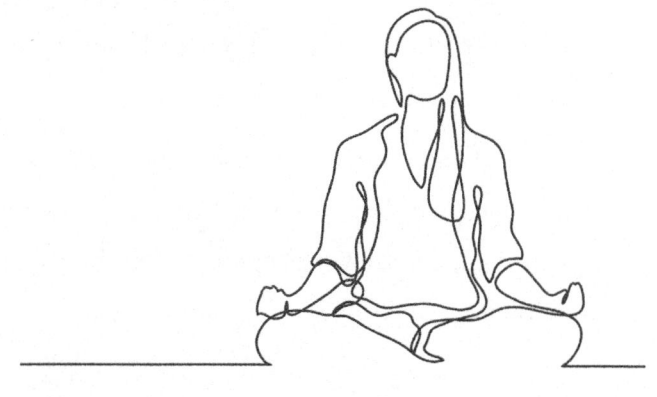

3 Types of Rest to Restore You to a Full Charge:

1. <u>Rest After Exercise:</u> Physical Rest: After a workout, your muscles need time to recover. Adequate physical rest involves allowing your body to relax and repair itself. This can include avoiding intense workouts targeting the same muscle groups for at least 48 hours, especially after strength training.

Sleep: Quality sleep is crucial for post-exercise recovery. Aim for 7-9 hours of restful sleep to support muscle repair, hormone production, and overall recovery.

Hydration and Nutrition: Proper hydration and balanced nutrition play a vital role in recovery. Ensure you're replenishing lost fluids and consuming a mix of macronutrients (protein, carbohydrates, and healthy fats) to aid in muscle recovery.

2. <u>Rest When You're Sick:</u> Physical Rest: When you're sick, your body's immune system is working hard to fight off illness. Physical rest involves avoiding strenuous activities to allow your immune system to focus on healing. Gentle, low-intensity movements like walking may be beneficial if your body feels up to it.

Sleep: Illness can disrupt sleep patterns, but restorative sleep is essential for recovery. Listen to your body and allow yourself extra sleep as needed to support the healing process.

Hydration and Nutrition: Stay hydrated and focus on nutrient-dense foods that provide vitamins and minerals to support your immune system. Sometimes, your appetite might be reduced, so aim for easily digestible options.

3. <u>Rest After a Stressful Period</u>: Mental Rest: After a stressful period, your mind may need a break. Engage in activities that promote relaxation and mindfulness, such as meditation, deep breathing, or simply spending time in nature.

Social Rest: If your stress was related to social interactions or demands, consider spending time with supportive friends and family, or even taking a break from social commitments.

Sleep: Sleep is vital for mental and emotional well-being. Adequate sleep helps regulate mood and reduces stress levels. Ensure you get enough sleep to feel refreshed and rejuvenated.

Recreational Activities: Engage in hobbies or activities that bring you joy and help take your mind off stress. Whether it's reading, painting, or gardening, leisure activities can provide a sense of mental renewal.

Remember that everyone's needs are unique, and it's essential to listen to your body and mind. Pay attention to how you feel and adjust your rest strategies accordingly. In some cases, seeking guidance from healthcare professionals, such as a doctor or a registered dietitian, can help you determine the appropriate kind of rest based on your individual circumstances and needs. Rest is a crucial component of self-care, contributing to your overall health, recovery, and resilience.

The Empowering Nap

Afternoon naps, also known as power naps or cat naps, have been shown to have positive effects on energy levels, alertness, and NuCalm and Calm are examples of technology-based tools designed to promote relaxation, reduce stress, and enhance overall well-being.

Presctiption Strength

These technologies utilize various approaches, such as neurostimulation, biofeedback, and guided meditation, to achieve their goals. While specific long-term benefits may vary depending on individual use and circumstances, here are some potential long-term benefits of using technologies like NuCalm and Calm.

Stress Reduction: Both NuCalm and Calm employ techniques that help reduce stress levels by calming the nervous system and promoting relaxation. Consistent use of these technologies over time can lead to decreased stress and a greater ability to manage daily challenges.

Improved Sleep Quality: Stress and anxiety can negatively impact sleep. Technologies like Calm often include guided meditation and relaxation exercises that can improve sleep quality over time by promoting a calm and restful state of mind.

Enhanced Mental Clarity and Focus: Regular practice with these technologies may lead to improved mental clarity and focus. Reduced stress and a clearer mind can enhance cognitive function and productivity in daily activities.

Mindfulness and Self-Awareness: Many relaxation and meditation techniques included in these technologies promote mindfulness and self-awareness. Over time, increased mindfulness can lead to better emotional regulation and a deeper understanding of one's thoughts and feelings.

Emotional Well-Being: NuCalm and Calm often include content aimed at enhancing emotional well-being, such as guided meditation for anxiety, gratitude exercises, and practices for cultivating positive emotions. These tools can contribute to long-term emotional resilience and a more positive outlook on life.

Reduced Physical Symptoms of Stress: Chronic stress can manifest in physical symptoms such as muscle tension, headaches, and gastrointestinal issues. The relaxation techniques used in these technologies may help alleviate these symptoms over time.

Heart Health: Stress management techniques have been linked to improved heart health by reducing blood pressure and promoting overall cardiovascular well-being.

Resilience to Future Stressors: Learning effective stress reduction techniques through technologies like NuCalm and Calm can equip individuals with skills to manage stress more effectively when faced with future challenges.

Long-Term Relaxation Habits: Consistently using these technologies can help individuals establish healthy relaxation habits, leading to a proactive approach to stress management and self-care.

Presctiption Strength

Psychological and Emotional Benefits: Engaging with calming technologies can contribute to a sense of well-being, emotional balance, and a greater capacity to cope with life's ups and downs.

It's important to note that while technology-based relaxation tools can offer many potential benefits, they are most effective when used as part of a holistic approach to well-being. Combining their use with other lifestyle factors such as a balanced diet, regular exercise, sufficient sleep, and social support can amplify the positive impact on overall health and wellness.

As with any wellness practice, individual experiences may vary, and it's advisable to consult with a healthcare professional if you have specific health concerns.

Cognitive Performance: Numerous studies have investigated the impact of short naps on productivity and overall well-being.

Here are some key findings related to improved productivity when afternoon naps are utilized to boost energy levels:

Enhanced Alertness and Cognitive Function: Research has consistently shown that short naps (typically lasting 10 to 30 minutes) can lead to improved alertness, concentration, and cognitive function. These benefits can translate to increased productivity and better performance in tasks requiring attention and focus.

Improved Memory and Learning: Napping has been linked to better memory consolidation and learning. Studies have found that a nap following a learning session can enhance the retention of newly acquired information, which can be especially beneficial for students and professionals.

Mood Enhancement: Afternoon naps have been associated with improved mood and decreased feelings of irritability and fatigue. A more positive mood can contribute to a better work environment and increased productivity.

Reduced Fatigue and Sleepiness: Napping can help counteract the natural drop in energy levels that often occurs in the afternoon, particularly after lunch. By reducing fatigue and sleepiness, naps can help individuals maintain their focus and productivity throughout the day.

Creative Thinking: Some studies suggest that napping may enhance creative thinking and problem-solving abilities. A brief nap can provide a mental reset that allows individuals to approach challenges with a fresh perspective.

Physical and Psychological Well-Being: Napping can contribute to overall well-being by providing a brief period of rest and relaxation. Improved well-being can lead to better mental health and a more positive outlook, both of which can positively impact productivity.

Presctiption Strength

It's important to note that the effectiveness of afternoon naps in boosting productivity may vary depending on individual factors such as sleep habits, sleep needs, and the timing and duration of the nap. While short naps can be beneficial, longer naps (over 30 minutes) may lead to sleep inertia, which is a groggy feeling upon waking that can temporarily impair performance.

To make the most of afternoon naps for productivity:
- Keep naps short. Aim for around 10 to 30 minutes to avoid grogginess.
- Choose the right time. Napping in the mid-afternoon, typically between 2 p.m. and 3 p.m., aligns with the body's natural circadian rhythm.
- Create a conducive environment. Find a quiet, dark, and comfortable space for napping.

*Pay attention to how naps affect your energy levels and adjust the timing and duration to find what works best for you.

Overall, incorporating well-timed and appropriate afternoon naps into your routine can contribute to increased productivity, improved mood, and better

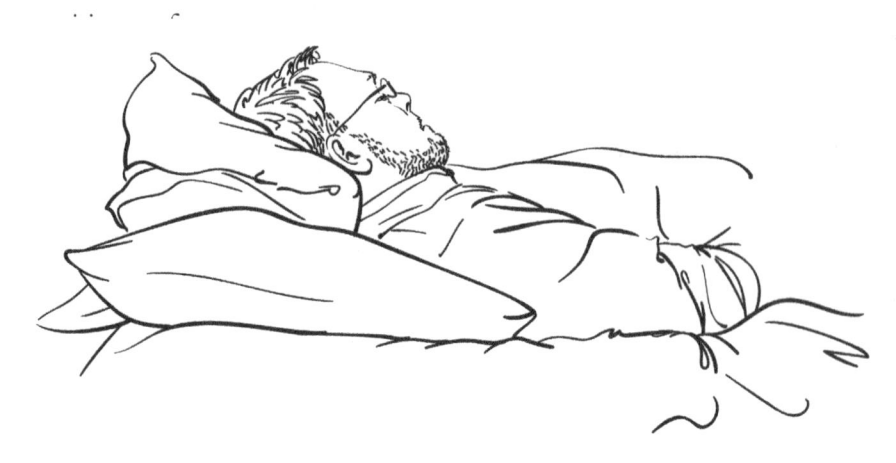

More Rest

Have a Sleep Rest Routine
1. Eating right throughout the day will also help you sleep better at night.
2. Getting at least 15 minutes of even light exercise, which could include brisk walking, will help your body feel more naturally tired at night.
3. Know Your Stimulants - Depending on how caffeine affects you, avoid it 7-10 hours before bedtime.
4. Know Your Bladder - Depending on your ability to "hold it," avoid drinking liquids 2-3 hours before sleep time.
5. Complete a Short Checklist - 5-10 minutes before bed consider a to do list that could include using the toilet, showering, brushing your teeth, reading something non stressful or reviewing a few things you are thankful for.

Pro Tips for Your Sleeping Space
1. The Darker the Better - From black-out shades on the windows to removing or covering anything that creates light in your sleeping area is important.
2. On the Cooler Side - Many experts will say to keep the room 65-69 degrees so that it's cold enough to have a blanket over you comfortably.
3. Covers with Weight - Using blankets that are heavy enough to create a certain amount of weight convering you is a form of pressure therapy helping you reach quality sleep.
4. Soft but Supportive Balance - When it comes to your pillow and your mattress, you will want soft but supportive, and don't forget the typical mattress is only good for 7-10 years.
5. Secure Your Space - Shut bedroom doors and closet doors to create a finite space that is closed up and feeling safe. Some people will even need windows locked up tight.

IF YOU CAN NOT *MEASURE IT,* YOU CAN NOT *IMPROVE IT.*

- LORD KELVIN

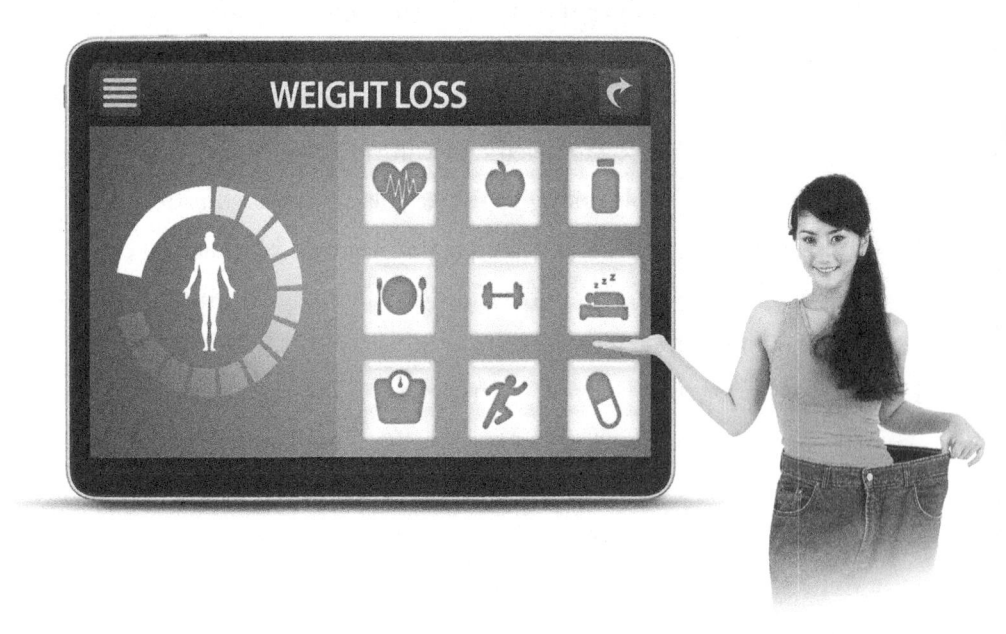

CHAPTER 8
Monitor with Technology

When it comes to your weight and, even more specifically your health, you need to use everything you have at your disposal. That's the same thinking we used to design our SimpleMD® 8 Pillars of Perpetual Health and Wellbeing. It's the epitome of using every weapon in the arsenal and every tool in the chest. This includes technology.

There's an expression, "You have to track it to crack it," which kind of goes with another one that says, "What gets measured gets improved." Whether it's personally or professionally, physical health or mental health, there is a need to know if we are progressing. Seeing results has a powerful effect on our attitude to endure more and go further.

Technology is probably the best way to track our vitals, our measurements, and, ultimately, our progress. This doesn't mean you need to stare at a scale every hour or even every day. Rather, it just means there's more than one way to gauge our body's health metrics.

Certainly, there is a wide range of technology available to help individuals monitor their sleep, measure heart rate, and manage exercise routines. Let's start with some of the technologies that exist and what data they can provide you with.

Presctiption Strength

Top 10 Techs that can Tell You About Yourself:

1. <u>Fitness Trackers</u> (e.g., Fitbit, Garmin, Apple Watch): These wearable devices provide comprehensive health tracking, including step counting, heart rate monitoring, sleep analysis, and workout metrics. They sync with your smartphone to provide real-time data and insights.

2. <u>Smartwatches</u> (e.g., Apple Watch, Samsung Galaxy Watch): In addition to fitness tracking features, smartwatches offer customizable apps, notifications, and built-in GPS. They can also monitor heart rate and sleep patterns.

3. <u>Sleep Tracking Devices</u> (e.g., Oura Ring, Withings Sleep Analyzer): These devices analyze sleep stages, track sleep duration, monitor sleep quality, and provide insights to improve sleep habits.

4. <u>Heart Rate Monitors</u> (e.g., Polar, Wahoo, Garmin): Wearable chest straps or wrist-based heart rate monitors help track your heart rate during workouts, providing accurate data to optimize exercise intensity.

5. <u>Pedometers and Step Counters</u> (e.g., Omron, Xiaomi Mi Band): Basic devices focused on counting steps and encouraging physical activity throughout the day.

6. <u>Smart Scales</u> (e.g., Withings Body+, Fitbit Aria): These scales not only measure weight but also provide additional data like body composition, muscle mass, and BMI. Some sync with fitness apps for comprehensive tracking.

Monitor with Technology

7. <u>Fitness Apps</u> (e.g., MyFitnessPal, Nike Training Club, Strava): These mobile applications allow you to log workouts, track nutrition, monitor progress, and set goals. Many integrate with wearable devices for seamless data syncing.

8. <u>Mobile Health Platforms</u> (e.g., Apple Health, Google Fit): These built-in smartphone apps consolidate health and fitness data from various sources, providing a holistic view of your well-being.

9. <u>Blood Pressure Monitors</u> (e.g., Omron, Withings): These devices measure blood pressure at home and can help you keep tabs on your cardiovascular health.

10. <u>Home Gym Tech</u> (e.g., Peloton, Mirror, Tonal): Interactive home fitness equipment that offers guided workouts, tracks performance, and adjusts resistance automatically.

*I'm not endorsing any one specific tech or brand at the moment, but I just wanted you to have powerful information and keep the attitude of using everything at your disposal.

Remember that while these technologies can provide valuable insights and motivation, they should complement a balanced approach to health and fitness, which includes proper nutrition, sleep, and regular physical activity. Before adopting any new technology or making significant changes to your exercise routine, it's a good idea to consult with a healthcare professional, especially if you have underlying health conditions.

Presctiption Strength

You can see a pattern or a common thread throughout these technologies of certain things that get tracked more than others. Let's look at that list as well.

Top 10 Health Metrics Worth Measuring:

1. <u>Heart Rate</u>: This can determine resting heart rate and, in theory, even when you sleep, as well as at what stage of sleep you're in and for how long. This reveals REM sleep, Deep sleep, and Light sleep. This information can even be used to give you a sleep score. In addition to resting and sleep, your rate can reveal when you're in various zones of cardio, like fat-burning zones and peak zones. This can lead to determining calories burned and the range of your heartbeats from completely resting to full exertion.

2. <u>Body Makeup</u>: Weight is only one way to determine your health but isn't necessarily the best way. Many of these scales and suits that exist today can also reveal bone density, total body water, and body fat percentage, which is probably the most helpful when determining if your diet provides you with positive results.

3. <u>Sleep Zones</u>: Know not just that you are sleeping but that you are getting enough Deep Sleep and REM sleep versus light sleep is important. More than a few devices will track this for you. Knowing the outcome can allow you to be more purposeful with your sleep strategies and methods. Plus, if you can see that you are getting relatively good sleep but still feel tired now, you can check something off the list as you work to determine how to raise your energy levels during the day.

Monitor with Technology

4. <u>Step Counters</u>: Knowing how many steps you take has become a good indicator of daily exercise, movement and blood circulation. The magic number seems to be 10,000 and we will discuss that more.

*Careful, some of these technologies that gamify things and make them fun can also be slightly addictive. You can find yourself constantly checking stats in an unhealthy way.

One good thing to gamify a little and track is steps. I know that if you are getting some good steps in, then several great things are happening in your body.

International Symbol and Sign of Health

In the pursuit of a healthier lifestyle, the concept of walking 10,000 steps a day has gained significant popularity. This daily step goal has become a symbol of physical activity and a cornerstone of fitness tracking. But how did this notion begin, and what does research tell us about its benefits?

Origins of the 10,000 Steps Goal: The origins of the 10,000 steps goal can be traced back to Japan in the 1960s. Dr. Yoshiro Hatano, a Japanese researcher, developed the concept of "manpo-kei," which translates to "10,000 steps meter" in English. Dr. Hatano's research aimed to find a simple and achievable way for individuals to engage in regular physical activity to improve their health. He chose the 10,000 steps figure based on his observations of average daily activity levels and their potential impact on cardiovascular health.

Presctiption Strength

Health Benefits of Walking 10,000 Steps a Day
There are quite a few benefits to putting in the steps:
- Cardiovascular Health - Regular walking can enhance heart health by improving blood circulation, reducing blood pressure, and lowering the risk of heart disease and stroke.
- Weight Management - Walking burns calories and contributes to weight loss or weight maintenance, aiding in achieving a healthy body weight.
- Bone Health - Weight-bearing activities like walking promote bone density, reducing the risk of osteoporosis and fractures.
- Mental Well-Being - Walking stimulates the release of endorphins, which can reduce stress, anxiety, and depression while enhancing mood and cognitive function.
- Diabetes Management - Walking helps regulate blood sugar levels, making it beneficial for managing and preventing type 2 diabetes.
- Joint Mobility - Walking is a low-impact exercise that improves joint flexibility and reduces the risk of joint-related issues.
- Longevity - Engaging in regular physical activity, such as walking 10,000 steps, has been associated with increased longevity and a higher quality of life in later years.

Research and Scientific Backing: Numerous studies have explored the health benefits of walking, including the 10,000 steps concept. Research has shown that walking can lead to improvements in cardiovascular fitness, weight control, metabolic health, mental well-being, and overall physical function.

While the specific number of steps might not be a one-size-fits-all prescription, the general idea of incorporating more movement into daily life has been widely embraced.

Keep it Moving Japanese Style

Moreover, advancements in wearable fitness trackers and smartphone apps have enabled individuals to monitor their step count and set achievable goals easily. Research has also focused on the feasibility and adherence to walking-based interventions, especially in sedentary populations. Walking is accessible, requires no special equipment, and can be adapted to various fitness levels, making it an attractive choice for promoting physical activity.

In conclusion, the concept of walking 10,000 steps a day has evolved from a simple idea to a globally recognized approach to improving health and well-being. While the specific step count may vary based on individual factors, the underlying principle of incorporating more movement into daily routines remains sound. Research continues to support the myriad benefits of walking, confirming its status as a valuable tool in the quest for a healthier and more active lifestyle.

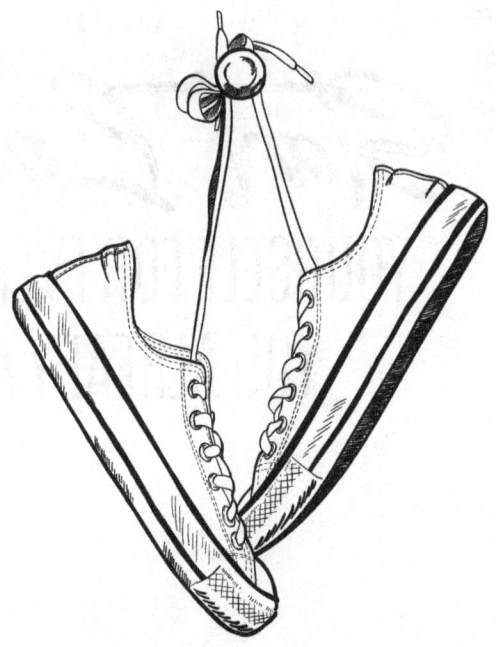

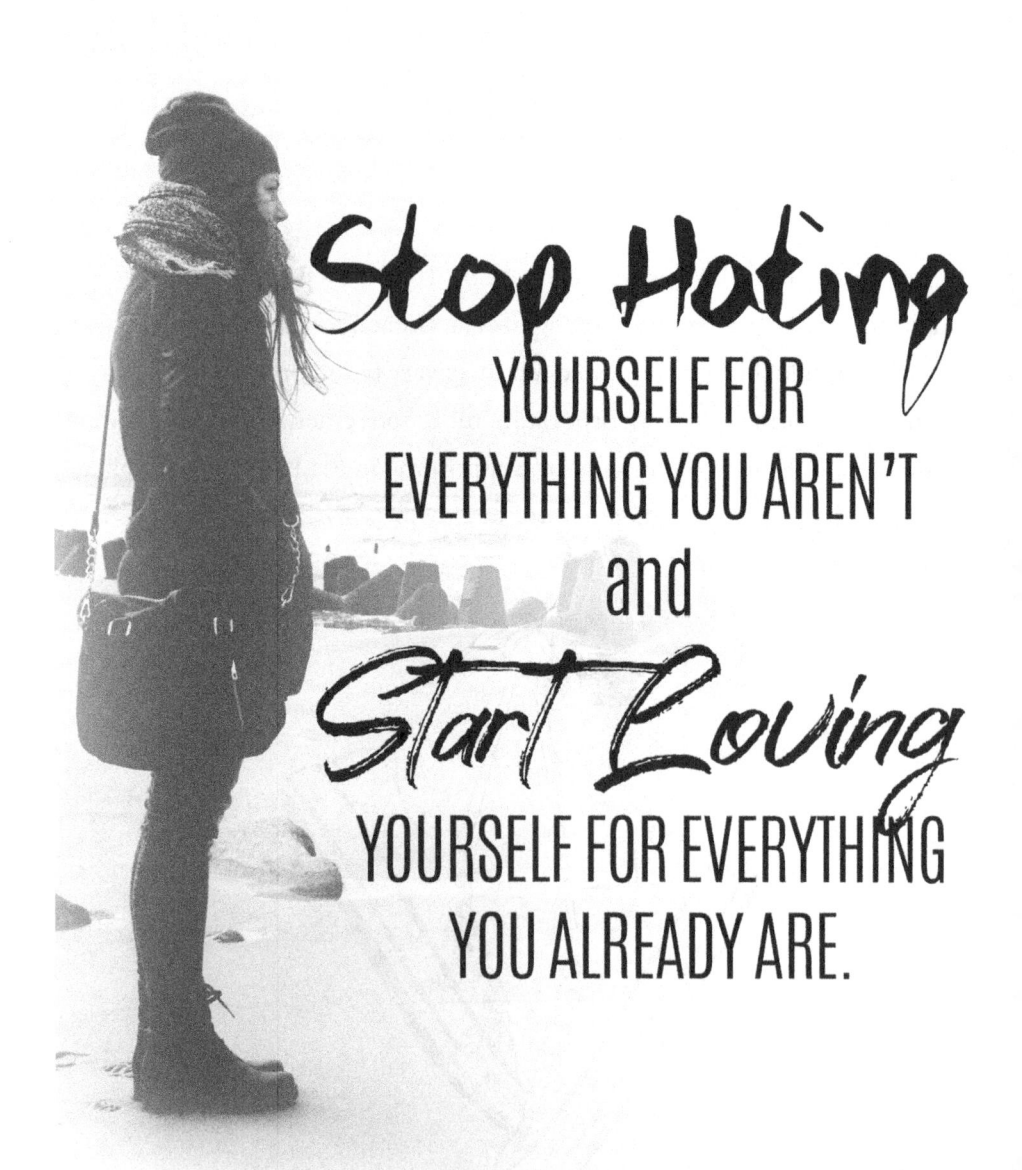

Stop Hating YOURSELF FOR EVERYTHING YOU AREN'T and *Start Loving* YOURSELF FOR EVERYTHING YOU ALREADY ARE.

CHAPTER 9
Master Your Emotions

If the most important pillar in the 8 Pillars of Perpetual Health and Wellbeing is to consume only healthy food, then it's worth noting that one of the biggest enemies of healthy eating is your emotions. Many people who struggle with weight and other health problems because of that weight do so because they are emotional eaters. They eat to feel good, to feel comfortable, and to connect emotionally with others.

On the surface, it doesn't sound so bad, I suppose. We form some of our best memories with our parents and families sharing meals. Whether you are sitting down at the table, lounging around a TV, or out at a restaurant, the subconscious bonding that happens during a shared meal is profound.

Birthdays, holidays, anniversaries, weekly dinners with extended family, nights out with co-workers or friends, and more all trigger a reprioritization of our goals, the lowering of our defenses, and an override button that drops us back into old patterns and habits.

It's Strong to Know Your Weaknesses

You need to be aware and conscious of your emotions. Knowing what triggers you and what your weaknesses are is important when it comes to keeping your commitments to lose weight and get healthy. Some of my friends can't go to sporting events while dieting. At least not for a little while. Others I know

Presctiption Strength

won't go out while getting back in shape. I even have a close friend who stopped working on the road traveling for business because staying healthy was just too hard living out of a suitcase in hotel rooms.

Unintended Parenting

Your mother telling you to finish your plate and not to waste food is often a tradition they came down from a time like the Great Depression when there was often not enough food to go round. These well-intended "force feedings" often did more harm than realized.

Another fun idea that has gone wrong is your mother or your father rewarding you as a child with candy, ice cream, and other sweets, not knowing how they were programming you, tying emotions to food.

Emotional eating refers to the act of consuming food in response to emotional triggers, feelings, or psychological states rather than in response to physical hunger. It involves using food as a way to cope with, suppress, or manage emotions, which can lead to overeating or consuming specific comfort foods. Emotional eating is often driven by a desire to alleviate negative emotions, seek comfort, or distract oneself from emotional distress.

Identifying an Emotional Eater

Eating When Not Hungry: Emotional eaters often eat even when they are not physically hungry. They may consume food out of boredom, sadness, stress, anxiety, or other emotional states.

Specific Food Cravings: Emotional eaters tend to have strong cravings for specific comfort foods, which are often high in sugar, fat, or carbohydrates. These foods are chosen for their ability to provide temporary emotional relief.

Sudden Urges to Eat: Emotional eating episodes may be triggered suddenly by an emotional event, stressor, or negative mood. The urge to eat can be intense and difficult to resist.

Mindless Eating: Emotional eaters may consume food mindlessly, without paying attention to portion sizes or taste. They might eat quickly and not fully savor the flavors of the food.

Emotional Triggers: Emotional eaters may eat in response to specific emotional triggers, such as stress, sadness, loneliness, anger, frustration, or boredom.

Lack of Physical Hunger Cues: Emotional eaters may have difficulty recognizing or distinguishing between physical hunger and emotional hunger. Physical hunger tends to be gradual and accompanied by physical cues like stomach growling.

Guilt and Regret: After an emotional eating episode, individuals may experience feelings of guilt, regret, or shame for consuming more food than they intended.

Pattern of Overeating: Emotional eating can become a pattern or habit, occurring regularly in response to emotional situations.

Presctiption Strength

Ways to Address Emotional Eating:

Mindful Eating: Practicing mindful eating involves paying full attention to the eating experience, savoring flavors, and being aware of hunger and fullness cues.

Emotion Regulation Techniques: Learn healthy ways to manage emotions, such as deep breathing, meditation, journaling, or engaging in hobbies you enjoy.

Seek Support: Reach out to friends, family, or a mental health professional to discuss your emotions and find healthier ways to cope.

Physical Activity: Engage in regular exercise, which can help improve mood and reduce stress without relying on food.

Identify Triggers: Become aware of situations, places, or emotions that trigger emotional eating and develop strategies to cope with them.

Nutrition Education: Learn about balanced nutrition and healthy eating habits to make informed food choices.

Create a Supportive Environment: Surround yourself with positive influences, and avoid keeping unhealthy comfort foods readily available.

Professional Help: If emotional eating becomes a significant concern or if it interferes with your well-being, consider seeking guidance from a registered dietitian, therapist, or counselor.

Remember that overcoming emotional eating is a journey, and it may involve trial and error to find the strategies that work best for you. It's important to approach the process with self-compassion and a willingness to address the underlying emotions that contribute to this behavior.

Sarah's Story *(Names have been fictionalized for patient privacy concerns)*
Once upon a time, in the small town of Brookville, there lived a vibrant and determined woman named Sarah. Sarah had struggled with obesity for most of her adult life and had reached a point where she knew she needed to make a change. She turned to her trusted primary care provider, Dr. Roberts, who let her know of his practice's new weight loss program called SimpleMD, with a revolutionary medically supervised treatment option – semaglutide, a GLP-1 agonist injection.

Sarah had always been a social butterfly, and her love for life often led her to enjoy evenings filled with laughter and glasses of wine. However, as she embarked on her journey with semaglutide, she noticed a remarkable shift in her food cravings and desires. Surprisingly, the medication had also had a profound impact on her relationship with alcohol.

In the early stages of her treatment, Sarah began to experience a newfound sense of fullness and reduced appetite. The constant cravings she once had for alcohol seemed to fade away. As she became more attuned to her body's needs and listened to its signals, the allure of alcohol gradually lost its grip on her.

Sarah's commitment to her health and weight loss goals grew stronger with each passing day. The positive changes she witnessed in her body and mindset fueled her determination to maintain her newfound lifestyle. She dedicated herself to regular exercise, balanced nutrition, and staying true to the guidelines set by Dr. Roberts and the help of her SimpleMD® Coach.

As the weeks turned into months, Sarah started noticing remarkable changes. The pounds began to melt away, and her confidence soared. She reached her goal weight, a milestone she had dreamt of for years. But it wasn't just the physical transformation that thrilled her; it was the newfound sense of empowerment and self-discovery.

Throughout her journey, Sarah had also discovered a deep appreciation for the clarity and mental focus she experienced without alcohol. She relished the mornings free from hangovers, allowing her to embrace each day with enthusiasm and productivity. She found solace in the natural high that came from taking care of her body and nourishing her spirit.

Sarah's decision to abstain from alcohol became a conscious choice, rooted in her unwavering commitment to her well-being. She realized that the joy she had once associated with drinking alcohol paled in comparison to the fulfillment she found in her healthier lifestyle.

Going Viral

Time passed, and Sarah's transformation became an inspiration to those around her. Her story spread throughout the community, motivating others to take charge of their health and make positive changes. She became an advocate for holistic well-being, sharing her experiences and encouraging others to explore the benefits of a life without excessive alcohol consumption.

Sarah's journey was not without challenges, but her unwavering determination and the support of her healthcare team helped her triumph over the obstacles along the way. She happily embraced her alcohol-free lifestyle, reveling in the freedom it offered her and the profound impact it had on her overall health and happiness.

As time went on, Sarah continued to thrive, never once feeling the need to reintroduce alcohol into her life. She cherished the clarity, energy, and zest for life that she had discovered through her journey with semaglutide and the lifestyle changes she had embraced with the SimpleMD® team by her side.

Sarah's story is a testament to the transformative power of making conscious choices and prioritizing one's health. It serves as a reminder that the pursuit of well-being is a personal journey, and each individual has the power to shape their destiny. With determination, team support, and a willingness to embrace change, Sarah not only achieved her goal weight but also found a renewed sense of purpose and contentment that should guide her throughout her life.

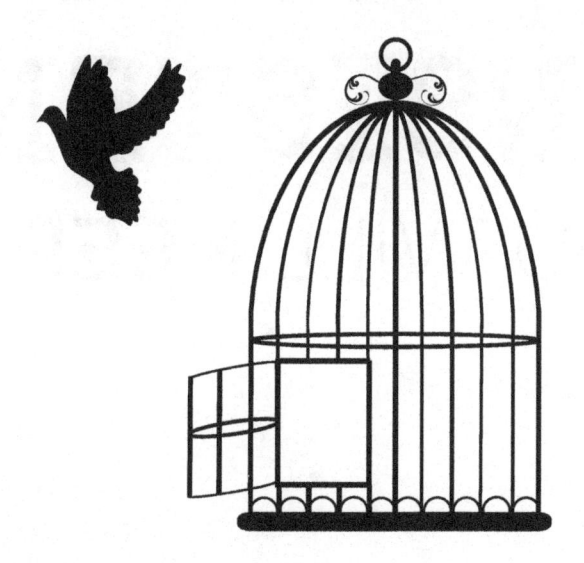

IF **YOU** ARE
PERSISTENT,
YOU WILL **GET IT**.

◇

IF **YOU** ARE
CONSISTENT,
YOU WILL **KEEP IT**.

CHAPTER 10
Make Healthy Habits

Following this Prescription Strength program can easily result in noticeable weight loss in weeks, not months. This is the start of your "reset," changing your individual weight set point on a molecular level. This sets into motion so many health benefits and even augments future capacity to lose even more weight.

You might have skipped right to this chapter to get to the good stuff! In previous chapters, I've worked to make the case that the Mediterranean Lifestyle, coupled with the proper use of GLP-1 agonists—such as Ozempic, Wegovy, Mounjaro and Rybelsus—and lifestyle changes, has ushered in the most exciting developments in weight loss and healthy living I've ever seen. People who adopt this lifestyle pattern live longer, with less disease and greater health than virtually any other people on the globe.

It's time to turn all this knowledge into practical, day-to-day action. I often tell people that, unless they are willing to move to some of the blue zones of southern Italy, they'll have to find a way to make their commitment to these changes in their actual, hectic, American lives. And that's what this chapter is all about, so don't worry: I'm not going to advise that you cut back hours in the office, learn how to cook like an Italian grandmother, and source your fresh ingredients every morning from a village market. Instead, this is all about combining modern science with the age-old wisdom of the Mediterranean Lifestyle to work for you, in your current life. This is why we created SimpleMD®, and I am confident you'll see that it really can be fast and simple.

Presctiption Strength

Dieting vs. Lifestyle

Before I get started, I think it's important to touch a little bit on the difference between a diet and making a positive lifestyle change. Diets are something of a national obsession. Depending on which statistics you look at, as many as one in five Americans say they are on a diet on any given day, with most of them aiming to lose about twenty pounds. This means every day, you can find tens of millions of Americans following whatever rules their weight-loss plan describes. They might be weighing foods, counting calories, figuring out food scores, cutting out whole food groups, or living on concoctions that came from our ever-more-popular juicers.

Unfortunately, research has also shown that the vast majority of these diets will fail. These numbers are even harder to pin down, but it's not uncommon to read that more than 90 percent of dieters will ultimately gain back any weight they lost. So, what's my point? Simple: I am not advocating a "diet." Rather, I'm advocating healthy habits.

Lifestyle = Habit

We prescribe attitudes, approaches, and actions that lead to habit. We prescribe FDA-approved medications that will help you heal with healthy habits. We prescribe consistency that leads to habits, so you don't always have to have so much willpower and discipline. When your habits are healthy, your lifestyle automatically leads you in the right direction. This is a prescription of wins that lead to positive forward momentum that becomes not only sustainable but unstoppable.

Make Healthy Habits

A Few More SimpleMD® Philosophies

1. You are not dieting, rather you are creating a new weight set point.
2. You can and should enjoy—really enjoy—the food you eat!
3. You can easily create a lifestyle of positive habits!

You'll soon see that everything that I recommend falls in line with this philosophy. You don't need to count calories. If you like to cook, that's great—but if you don't, there's no reason to be stuck in the kitchen every day making every meal from scratch and portioning it out in little plastic containers. Success will come from understanding and counteracting the forces that got you there. In fact, you will probably feel better than ever before, while losing weight and making your doctor very happy during your checkups!

Traditionally, the first step in making any lifestyle change is the hardest—but that's not necessarily true any longer. Thanks to the GLP-1s, making those first changes to your diet and lifestyle is easier than ever. I've seen it myself: once the weekly injections take effect, your appetite melts away. The cravings and compulsions that characterize early-stage lifestyle changes and diets are absent. This kickstart to your program opens a door to making a truly healthy lifestyle change that will help you lose weight, feel better, reduce your risk of disease, and live longer.

Although I discussed the benefits of the revolutionary new prescription drugs, when re-setting your weight set point, ultimately, you will need a dietary regimen for the long term. Thus, for some patients who only have a few pounds to lose, our maximized mealtime and Mediterranean Lifestyle program might be enough for us to prescribe. For others who require more weight loss, a doctor can prescribe medications that are a very useful bridge to reset their biology.

Presctiption Strength

Relatively Easy is Different Than Easy

This doesn't mean you won't have hard days—even with help, making big changes is hard. But remember that no failure is permanent. If you have a bad day and slip back into older eating patterns, don't dwell on it! Tomorrow is another day so that you can start again. Guilt and self-reproach are negative influences that will try to knock you off your new program.

Your Relationship with Food Must Change

Medications are a key part of our approach, but long-term change also means making lifestyle changes that will outlast your GLP-1 prescription, including rethinking your approach to food. However, before we get into the food program itself, it's time to go into detail about Maximized Mealtime™.

In general, I've found two approaches that will work for most people. The first is commonly called intermittent fasting, or time-restricted eating. All of these things are habits that make the lifestyle, or a lifestyle made up of healthy habits.

The SimpleMD® Healthy Habits are:

1. No Eating After Dinner and only water or decaffeinated beverages at night.

2. Get Eight Hours Of Sleep. If your sleep is interrupted for some reason, do not eat! This can be hard at first, but it gets easier over time, and the medications can help.

3. For Maximum Weight Loss, consume only water and tea or coffee for the first four hours after you wake up. Skipping breakfast can be hard for some people, but again, medications can help blunt hunger/cravings. If you drink tea or coffee, avoid milk and sugar. You can use artificial sweeteners or a small amount of low-fat dairy.

4. <u>For Moderate Weight Loss,</u> limit yourself to three hundred calories in the first four hours. I suggest a variety of snack-sized Mediterranean Lifestyle options. The SimpleMD® bars are a useful substitute here (one to two bars in the morning).

5. <u>To Compensate For Eating Less Fiber</u>, I often recommend taking a light fiber supplement like Metamucil in the morning. I particularly enjoy the orange-flavored psyllium version that comes in convenient single-use packets in case I need it on the go. This is optional as everyone's digestive capacity and needs are a bit different. Eat your first meal after the four hours have passed. Enjoy a typical Mediterranean Lifestyle meal. Don't worry about counting calories or restricting any particular type of food, but be mindful and enjoy a single portion. Many patients choose to begin the eating period with a light Mediterranean Lifestyle snack or a bar to help them from overeating their first meal of the day. Those on the medications often solely rely on a Mediterranean Lifestyle snack or bar.

6. <u>Drink A Lot Of Water!</u> Water is particularly important in the first four hours. Water helps with overall digestion as well as satiety and can even reduce side effects if you're on a GLP-1 agonist.

7. <u>Enjoy Dinner In The Early Evening</u>. Once again, many patients sub-in a Mediterranean Lifestyle snack or bar. If you prepare food, however, don't worry about counting calories for this meal either. Just stick to the Mediterranean Lifestyle principles. You can also enjoy a light dessert. Some patients warm up a bar for ten seconds in a microwave and enjoy it with some noncaffeinated tea. This is a great way to begin the fasting period.

Presctiption Strength

Patients on the maintenance phase of their weight loss, or those who are starting the program without the help of medications, often report having a Mediterranean Lifestyle snack or a bar later at night as a healthier alternative that doesn't seem to set them back too much in their weight loss goals.

Cruise Control

Patients on the maintenance phase of their weight loss, or those who are starting the program without the help of medications, often report having a Mediterranean Lifestyle snack or a bar later at night as a healthier alternative that doesn't seem to set them back too much in their weight loss goals.

If you follow the pillars and principles, and keep in mind that minor indiscretions are not likely to derail your progress, drink more water if you make a mistake and overeat. Just have moderation with your moderation because it is a slippery slope. You will succeed in the long run and must keep that in mind at all times!

This pattern is best if you can stick to it seven days a week. For some patients, however, a "cheat day" is too important to skip. This hasn't been a problem, and for some people, it actually seems to be helpful for overall weight loss goals. If you're one of these people, go ahead and choose to take the occasional cheat day. Just get back on the regular program the next day.

If you're following this schedule, alcohol should be avoided as much as possible. There are many reasons for this, including empty calories, increased hunger, the dehydrating effects of alcohol, etc. However, if they do this in moderation (once or twice per week with one or two glasses of wine maximum), many have been able to continue the benefits of time-restricted eating and the Mediterranean Lifestyle.

Me with Weight Loss Medication and Alcohol

My personal experience was that drinking was undesirable during the GLP-1 initiation phase. Thus, my recommendation is to try to avoid alcohol while trying to reach your weight loss goals for optimal results.

When it comes to time-restricted eating, if it's too much at first, you can instead eat four or five small meals a day. Each meal will be 200–400 calories and should follow the Mediterranean Lifestyle approach, focusing on healthy vegetables and fats. If you prefer this approach, you may swap bars for one or two of your meals.

Make Your Meals Mediterranean

This is the fun part! Preparing meals should be a pleasure, almost as much as actually eating them. Above all, the Mediterranean Lifestyle is delicious.

Here are 10 Habits to Help Starters:

1. Eat fresh fruit or vegetables at every meal, including breakfast.
2. Enjoy unlimited quantities of green, leafy vegetables.
3. Aim to eat a wide variety of colorful vegetables and fruits.
4. Consume EVOO with at least one meal every day, but two or more is better.
5. All grains should be whole grains.

Presctiption Strength

6. Seafood should be your main source of protein.
7. Limit your intake of red meat.
8. Dairy food, especially cheese, should be eaten in limited quantities and not daily. Greek yogurt is the preferred form of dairy, as it contains lots of beneficial bacteria that help digestion.
9. Limit sweets and desserts.
10. Limit your intake of alcohol.

Hopefully, you can see how much variety is possible when you eat like this. You have permission to eat unlimited and healthy vegetables and fruits, plus a whole world of whole grains and seafood. Eating should be something you enjoy.

The medication will help you be disciplined, but the truth is you most likely won't think about food all that much when using prescription strength GLP-1's. It's during that time you get used to patterns, rituals, and routines that can more easily continue when you no longer take the medications. These habits can almost replace willpower in a sense. Get used to a lifestyle of loving your body more than loving food.

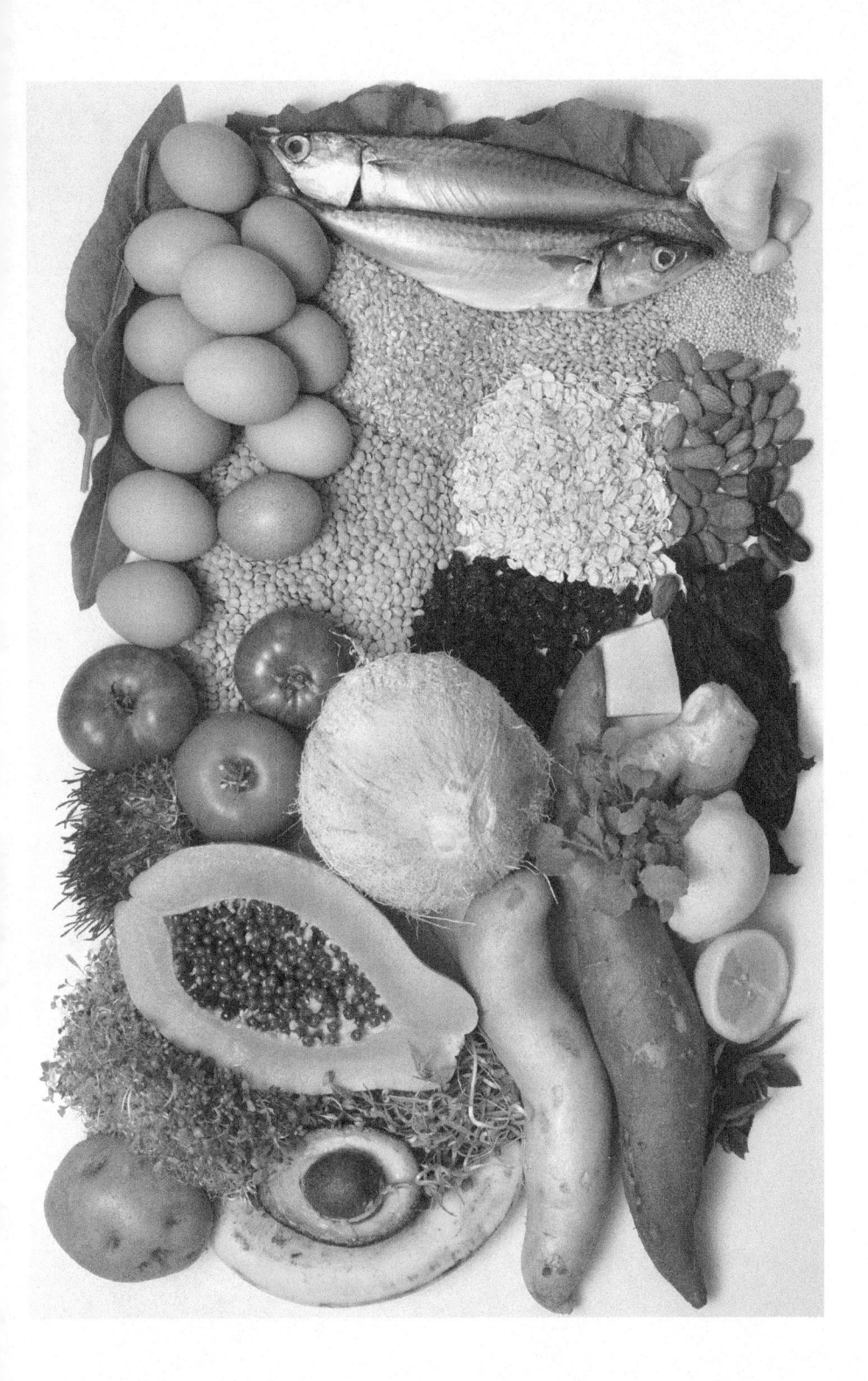

PART 4
Teamwork

Incoming call...

Your Dreams
are calling you

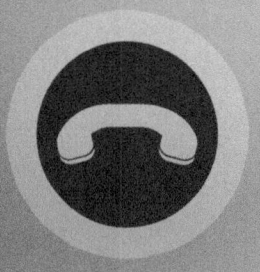

Decline   Accept

CHAPTER 11
Building Your Dream Team

You're going to want some key people in your corner. SimpleMD® has approved clinicians, physicians and coaches/concierges to help you along your way, but this might only be the core team. Your team could include fitness trainers, good friends with similar health goals, certified mentors and more.

You're going to end almost where you started. What are your goals? What do you want to do with all this extra energy you will have? Are you looking to be more active outside, travel or even compete at something? These things can also determine your team.

Team support is immensely valuable for helping individuals accomplish their goals. The presence of a supportive team can have a profound impact on an individual's motivation, progress, and overall success in reaching their objectives.

Here's the value of team support in achieving personal and professional goals:

Motivation and Encouragement: A supportive team provides motivation by cheering you on, celebrating your achievements, and offering words of encouragement during challenges. This positive reinforcement can boost your confidence and determination.

Presctiption Strength

Accountability: When you share your goals with a team, you become more accountable for your progress. Knowing that others are aware of your goals encourages you to stay on track and follow through on your commitments.

Collaborative Problem-Solving: Team members can offer different perspectives and ideas to help you overcome obstacles. Collaborative problem-solving often results in innovative solutions that you might not have thought of on your own.

Skill and Knowledge Sharing: Team members might have skills and knowledge that complement your own. This sharing of expertise can accelerate your learning and help you develop new competencies.

Increased Resources: A team brings together a variety of resources, including information, tools, connections, and experiences. These resources can provide valuable insights and shortcuts to achieving your goals.

Feedback and Improvement: Constructive feedback from team members can help you identify areas for improvement. Their insights can guide you toward refining your strategies and methods.

Networking and Connections: A team often includes individuals from diverse backgrounds and industries. Building relationships within the team can expand your network and open doors to new opportunities.

Reduced Stress and Pressure: The support of a team can alleviate stress by distributing the workload and providing emotional support. This can prevent burnout and help you maintain a healthier work-life balance.

Learning from Others' Experiences: Team members may have faced similar challenges in the past and can share their experiences, lessons learned, and strategies for overcoming obstacles.

Boosted Confidence: Knowing that you have a team backing you can boost your confidence. Their belief in your abilities can help you overcome self-doubt and take on more ambitious goals.

Shared Celebrations: Achieving goals becomes more meaningful when you can celebrate with your team. Sharing successes enhances the sense of accomplishment and strengthens team cohesion.

Empowerment to Take Risks: With team support, you may feel more empowered to take calculated risks, knowing that you have a safety net of support if things don't go as planned.

Continuous Learning Environment: Interacting with team members exposes you to different viewpoints, skills, and experiences, fostering continuous learning and personal growth.

Long-Term Commitment: A team's support is not limited to a single goal; it can extend across various endeavors, creating a reliable source of encouragement and assistance as you work on different projects.

In summary, team support provides emotional, intellectual, and practical assistance that can accelerate your progress and enhance your chances of achieving your goals. The combined efforts, resources, and encouragement from a supportive team can make your journey more enjoyable and fruitful.

Presctiption Strength

Creating a supportive team to help someone struggling with weight loss requires a compassionate and understanding approach. The dynamics of such a team should focus on providing encouragement, accountability, knowledge, and emotional support.

Here's what makes a good team when it comes to helping someone with weight loss:

Empathy and Non-Judgment: A good team starts with empathy and a non-judgmental attitude. Members should be understanding of the struggles the individual is facing and create a safe space for them to share their challenges.

Positive Reinforcement: Encouragement and positive reinforcement are essential. Team members should offer praise and celebrate even small achievements, fostering a sense of accomplishment and motivation.

Accountability Partners: Having accountability partners within the team can help the individual stay on track. Regular check-ins and discussions about progress can keep them accountable for their actions.

Nutritional Knowledge: Team members with knowledge about nutrition can provide guidance on healthy eating habits, meal planning, and portion control. This education helps the individual make informed choices.

Fitness and Exercise Support: If possible, including members who are knowledgeable about fitness and exercise can provide guidance on workout routines and activities that align with the individual's goals.

Supportive Environment: The team should foster a supportive environment where the individual feels comfortable discussing challenges and setbacks. This can prevent feelings of isolation and help them stay motivated.

Sharing Success Stories: Team members can share their own weight loss or health improvement stories to inspire and demonstrate that change is possible with determination.

Goal Setting and Tracking: The team can help the individual set achievable goals and track progress. This sense of accomplishment reinforces their commitment to their weight loss journey.

Healthy Lifestyle Tips: Team members can share practical tips for adopting a healthier lifestyle, such as managing stress, getting adequate sleep, and staying hydrated.

Cooking and Meal Preparation: If possible, team members who are skilled in cooking and meal preparation can provide ideas for nutritious and delicious recipes.

Mental and Emotional Support: Weight loss journeys often involve emotional challenges. Team members can offer emotional support, share coping strategies, and provide resources for managing stress and emotional eating.

Avoiding Triggers: Team members can help the individual identify triggers that lead to unhealthy eating habits and brainstorm strategies to avoid or manage those triggers.

Presctiption Strength

Progress Celebrations: Celebrate milestones and achievements together. Whether it's losing a certain amount of weight, completing a fitness milestone, or adopting a healthier habit, acknowledging progress boosts morale.

Flexible Approach: Recognize that weight loss journeys can be complex and require flexibility. The team should be adaptable to the individual's needs and progress pace.

Long-Term Commitment: Sustainable weight loss is a long-term goal. The team's support should extend beyond initial successes to ensure the individual maintains their progress.

Remember, the team's role is to provide guidance, support, and resources, but the individual's autonomy and agency in their weight loss journey are essential. The team should empower the individual to make choices that align with their goals and values while providing the tools they need to succeed.

SimpleMD® has an App that helps with finding like-minded people that has been shown to help in the medical weight loss journey. Studies have shown that a person's social surroundings can have a positive (or negative) effect on the amount of weight that is lost. So, we have designed a special App that allow selective social communication with others going through a similar journey.

Building Your Dream Team

Now the Medical Weight Loss Dream Team is in place. It is up to you to take your rightful place within it and enjoy the ride.

The best place to start building *your* team to meet your health goals is at SimpleMD.com

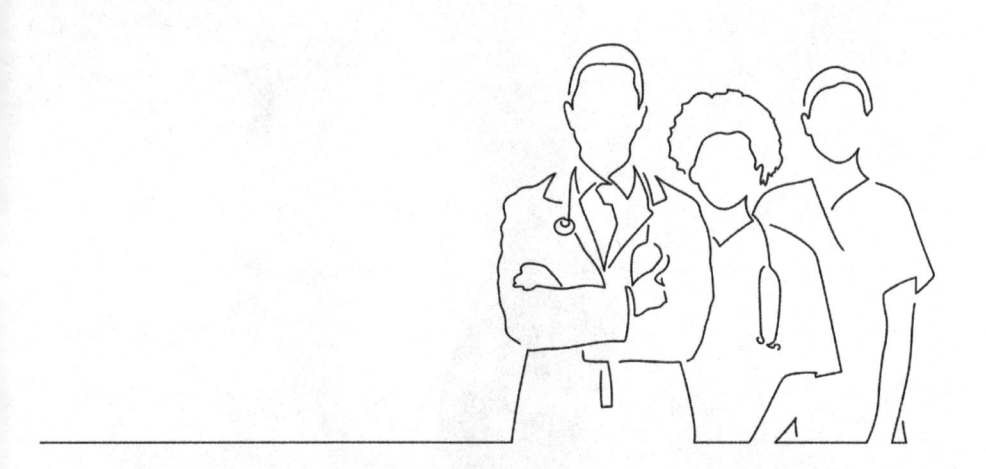

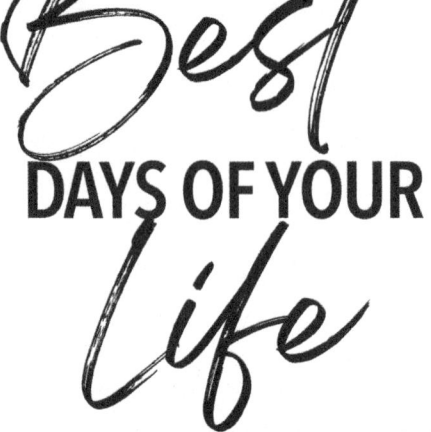

SOME OF THE *Best* DAYS OF YOUR *Life* HAVEN'T HAPPENED *Yet*...

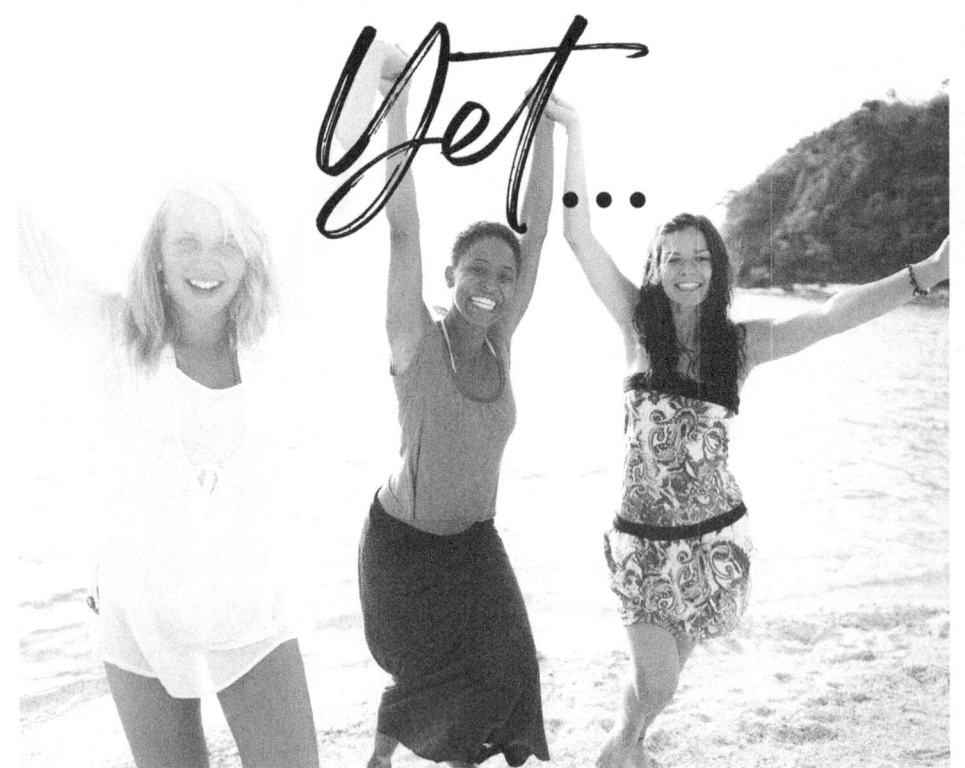

CHAPTER 12
Leveling Up

You may not be ready for this section. It's beyond the beginning and really for you to revisit once you got some real positive momentum and some fairly solidified healthy habits. This is an area we send people to as we see them advance with confidence.

This might be the more fun and fulfilling part because it's a place to think about life, legacy, and significance. If you think about Maslow's Hierarchy of Needs, which is essentially this triangle it starts at the bottom, where an individual is looking for more of the basic day to day needs of food and shelter and moves up from there with the top being a place of self-actualization.

It's only once we leave behind more of our distractions and addictions that we have the health and well-being to really be at full strength to discover what matters most to us. This isn't to say we all want to take over the world and or accomplish some monumental achievement rather it's to say that it's at this point and time you are at least able to consider what time and freedom from poor health and bad food might open up for you.

This freedom could be more time with your friends, family, and loved ones. It might mean you are writing your own book, you are taking that dream vacation, you are taking that painting class or dance class. Maybe it's time for you to start that side hustle or a new business altogether. Whatever it is, it takes confidence, energy, and belief in yourself.

Presctiption Strength

If you can take control of your weight and your health honestly, you can do just about anything. In some ways, this chapter is about the power of possibilities and opening yourself up to them. After all, you can't even dream of something that you don't even know exists, let alone find possible.

The time of leveling up and riding the wave of momentum happens when you take control of your health and your life. It's amazing the confidence you have when you feel good about yourself and you have the energy to put in the effort it takes to go to the next level.

This is a powerful place to be.

From Concern to Conviction: John's Transformation with Life-changing Medications

Disclaimer: The following story(s) is a fictionalized account inspired by real occurrences and patients within the healthcare field. The details have been altered to protect patient privacy and confidentiality.

In a quiet neighborhood, John, a talented statistician, found himself caught in the web of his family's history of obesity-related complications. With five siblings and parents who had experienced severe health issues due to obesity, John knew he had to take action. Though initially hesitant about taking medications, he eventually recognized that the potential benefits far outweighed any unknown risks. This fictionalized tale showcases John's journey of transformation and highlights the profound impact of these new medications.

At 38 years old, John was all too familiar with the devastating consequences of obesity. Witnessing his siblings and parents suffer from a range of health complications, including arthritis, lymphedema, sleep apnea, high cholesterol, high blood pressure, and inflammation, filled him with deep concern. Determined to break the cycle and regain control of his own health, John sought medical guidance.

With the support of his healthcare team, John made an informed decision to embark on a medication-assisted weight loss journey. Though initially apprehensive, he realized that the potential benefits of the new medications far exceeded any perceived risks. He acknowledged the importance of taking proactive steps to improve his health and break the familial pattern of obesity-related complications.

As the months passed, John's commitment and perseverance paid off in remarkable ways. The scale revealed a staggering weight loss of 130 pounds, bringing him to his goal weight. The positive changes extended far beyond his appearance. John experienced a complete transformation in his overall health and well-being.

The disappearance of his excess weight alleviated the burden on his joints, relieving him of the pain caused by arthritis. The once-present lymphedema, a condition that had hindered his mobility, diminished significantly. With the weight loss, John's sleep apnea symptoms vanished, allowing him to enjoy restful nights and wake up feeling refreshed and energized.

John's dedication to his weight loss journey also yielded incredible improvements in his cardiovascular health. His high cholesterol and high blood pressure markers normalized, reducing his risk of heart disease and related complications. Additionally, blood markers for inflammation showed a significant reduction, further mitigating his risk factors for other deadly diseases.

Empowered by his life-changing results, John became a passionate advocate for the benefits of these new medications. He recognized that the risk-benefit ratio was undeniably justified, given the remarkable improvements he experienced in his health and quality of life. John's conviction stemmed from his own transformative journey and the positive impact it had on his well-being. John is now training for his second half marathon and even more importantly, his monthly hikes with his kids have not only crated memories that will last a lifetime but have also broken the cycle of poor family fitness putting his loved ones at risk.

The Power of Support: Amanda's Journey to Sustainable Wellness with her SimpleMD® Team

In the vibrant city of Vitalityville, a remarkable woman named Amanda embarked on a life-changing journey to transform her health and well-being. With the unwavering support and guidance of her dedicated SimpleMD® healthcare team, Amanda not only achieved her weight loss goals but also discovered the power of coaching in sustaining her progress and embracing a healthier lifestyle

.

Amanda's journey began when she sought the expertise of her SimpleMD® healthcare team, who recognized her determination and commitment to her well-being. Together, they devised a comprehensive plan tailored to Amanda's unique needs and goals. The team provided invaluable support, combining their medical knowledge with compassionate coaching to empower Amanda throughout her transformation.

Through the prescribed GLP1 medications, Amanda experienced a rapid and significant weight loss, shedding an impressive 70 pounds in just four months. However, the journey did not end there. Recognizing the challenges of long-term maintenance, the SimpleMD® team played a crucial role in designing a personalized plan to ensure Amanda's continued success.

The coaching aspect of the SimpleMD® program proved to be a game-changer for Amanda. Regular communication with her healthcare team allowed her to discuss her progress, address challenges, and receive guidance on making sustainable lifestyle choices. They celebrated her achievements and provided gentle course corrections when needed, guiding her toward optimal health. The SimpleMD® App helped her to have private and useful contact with her Coach as well as mark her progress.

As Amanda transitioned into the maintenance phase, her SimpleMD® team remained by her side, offering ongoing support and encouragement. They reminded her of the importance of maintaining a healthy mindset and provided strategies to overcome any obstacles that came her way. Through their coaching, Amanda learned to navigate social situations, manage emotional eating, and develop a positive relationship with food.

The coaching sessions also focused on helping Amanda develop sustainable habits. The SimpleMD® team emphasized the importance of regular exercise

Presctiption Strength

and helped Amanda incorporate physical activity into her daily routine. They provided guidance on mindful movements, ensuring that Amanda's fitness journey aligned with her overall wellness goals.

A SimpleMD® Concierge

Amanda's SimpleMD® team understood the importance of addressing her emotional well-being as well. They encouraged her to practice self-care, engage in stress-management techniques, and foster a positive mindset. Through their guidance, Amanda developed resilience and learned to navigate life's challenges without resorting to emotional eating.

With the support of her SimpleMD® team, Amanda effortlessly maintained her weight loss and continued to enjoy optimal health. The team's knowledge, expertise, and genuine care empowered Amanda to embrace her new lifestyle with confidence and resilience. Their coaching had become an integral part of her journey, ensuring that Amanda never felt alone in her pursuit of wellness.

As Amanda's story continues to inspire, she remains forever grateful for her SimpleMD® team. Their coaching, encouragement, and expertise allowed her to achieve sustainable wellness, transform her life, and become an advocate for others embarking on their own journeys.

The power of support and coaching, as exemplified by her SimpleMD® team, forever remains at the heart of Amanda's triumphant transformation. Now Amanda is looking at joining the SimpleMD® team to help inspire others to do what she did. Her next level looks like passing the torch to others so that they might overcome obesity and achieve healthy living just like her.

Leveling Up

A Journey of Mindful Steps: Grace's Path to Effortless Weight Loss

In the serene town of Serenityville, a determined woman named Grace sought to transform her life and achieve her weight loss goals. With the guidance of her trusted SimpleMD® affiliated clinician, she discovered the power of mindful movements—a simple yet profound addition to her journey that would change her perception of exercise and pave the way to reaching her goal weight with unexpected ease.

During her consultation, Grace's clinician emphasized the importance of incorporating mindful movements into her weight loss routine. Intrigued by the concept, Grace delved deeper into understanding how simple actions could bring about significant changes in her body and mind. She soon realized that mindful movements were not just about physical activity, but also about cultivating a deeper connection with oneself and the present moment.

With this newfound knowledge, Grace decided to embrace a daily evening walk as her chosen form of mindful movement. Every day, as the sun dipped below the horizon, she would lace up her sneakers and embark on a tranquil journey through the neighborhood. However, this was no ordinary walk—it was a deliberate practice of mindfulness.

As Grace strolled along the familiar paths, she became fully present in each moment. She immersed herself in the sights, sounds, and sensations around her. She listened to the symphony of chirping birds, felt the gentle breeze caressing her skin, and marveled at the changing hues of the evening sky. She let go of worries and distractions, allowing her mind to find solace in the simplicity of the present moment.

With each step, Grace focused on her breath, syncing her inhalations and exhalations with the rhythm of her stride. She embraced the sensation of her feet connecting with the earth, grounding herself in the present. This mindful connection to her body and surroundings infused her walk with a sense of tranquility and purpose.

The effects of Grace's mindful walks extended far beyond the realm of physical activity. She discovered that this intentional practice had a profound impact on her overall well-being. The increased sense of calm and presence she experienced during her walks carried over into her daily life, allowing her to navigate stress and challenges with greater ease.

One unexpected benefit of Grace's mindful walks was the improvement in her sleep quality. The gentle exercise, combined with the mental clarity she achieved through mindfulness, helped her unwind and prepare her mind for restful sleep. Each night, as she laid her head on the pillow, she drifted off into a peaceful slumber, waking up refreshed and energized the next morning.

Over time, Grace's mindful walks became an integral part of her weight loss journey. With each stride, she shed not only physical weight but also mental and emotional burdens. The combination of mindful movement, improved sleep, and an overall sense of well-being led her to reach her goal weight with unexpected ease.

Leveling Up

In the tranquil town of Serenityville, Grace's journey became a symbol of the harmony that can be achieved through mindful movements. With SimpleMD®'s support and her unwavering commitment to self-care, Grace not only reached her goal weight but also discovered a profound sense of balance and inner peace.

Her story serves as a reminder that transformation can be found in the simplest of actions, and that by fostering a mindful connection to our bodies and the present moment, we can unlock the path to a more fulfilling and joyful life.

Grace now has 7-10 women (some pushing strollers) walking together 4 days a week in her neighborhood.

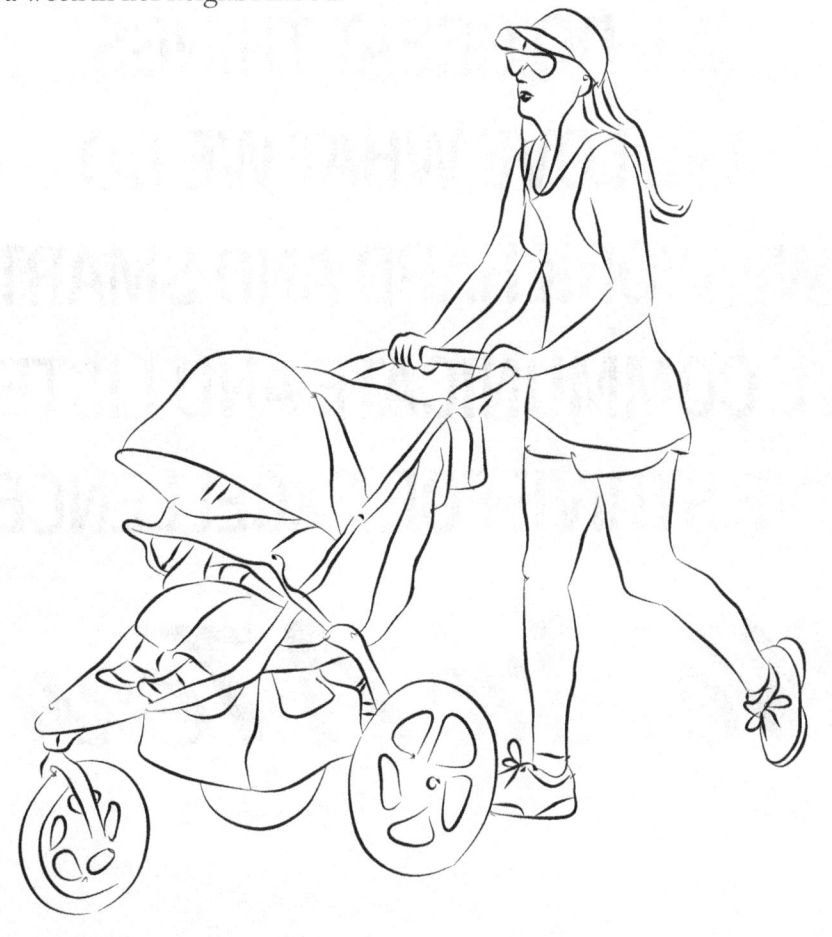

WE HAVE FUN
WE ARE HELPFUL
WE STAY POSITIVE
WE ARE RESPECTFUL
WE DO GREAT THINGS
WE LOVE WHAT WE DO
WE WORK HARD AND SMART
WE COMMUNICATE AND LISTEN
WE STRIVE FOR EXCELLENCE

We Are A Team

Epilogue
A Symphony and Dawn of a New Era

There is an untapped potential of breakthroughs in weight loss medications like the GLP-1's. In this ever-evolving landscape of healthcare, few discoveries have ignited as much hope and curiosity as GLP-1 medications. Known primarily for their transformative impact on diabetes and weight loss, these medications are the cornerstone of our mission at SimpleMD®. Yet, as we delve deeper into the labyrinth of human physiology, we're beginning to hear whispers of benefits that extend far beyond the realms of blood sugar and body mass.

The Symphony of Uncharted Benefits

While the scientific community is still in the early stages of understanding the full spectrum of GLP-1's potential, the voices of many patients are rising like a chorus, singing often unexpected praises these novel medications. Imagine a life where not only your physical health flourishes but your mental clarity sharpens like the blade of a samurai's sword. Picture a world where your cravings for alcohol and other addictions fade away like mist under the morning sun. Envision your skin glowing with the radiance of a thousand sunsets, and cellulite retreating like a defeated army. Even the dark clouds of depression and anxiety have been reported to scatter, making way for the light of emotional well-being.

Presctiption Strength

The Heart of the Matter

As if these anecdotal revelations weren't stirring enough, emerging research is adding robust notes to this symphony. Preliminary studies are painting an encouraging picture of GLP-1 medications as very beneficial to the heart, potentially becoming champions of cardiovascular vitality. In a world where heart disease plays the villain all too often, this is a melody of hope we cannot ignore. As a Board Certified Cardiovascular Specialist for 25 years privileged to treat thousands of heart and circulation patients through the years, this is simply music to my own ears and to our larger Cardiology community.

The Media's Discordant Tune

Yet, amidst this harmonious potential, the media often strikes a dissonant chord, amplifying the occasional negative side effect until it drowns out the myriad benefits. This cacophony can be overwhelming, leaving consumers adrift in a sea of confusion. We have come to realize that "if it bleeds it leads" in the media today. Nevertheless, responsible media tries to underscore the risk to benefit ratio that exists in any clinical innovation. I am hopeful that patient demand for a better, more effective treatment for unwanted weight gain, will ensure a fair duet between benefits and occasional risks, and not the salacious negative solo that sells advertisement but ultimately slows progress.

SimpleMD®: Your Conductor in the Orchestra of Health

This is where SimpleMD® steps onto the stage, baton in hand, ready to conduct this complex orchestra. We are committed to being an ongoing resource, a lighthouse in the storm, guiding you through the medical maze. We sift through the noise, separating fact from fiction so that you can embark on your medical weight loss journey with clarity and confidence.

Epilogue

We are pioneers, one of the first national companies to assemble a dream team of scientists, clinicians, educators, pharmacists, and most importantly, patients from around the globe. These are the voices that matter, the real-life experiences that enrich our understanding and fuel our mission.

The Future's Crescendo

As we look to the horizon, we stand ready for every advance, controversy, and breakthrough. We celebrate not just the scientific milestones but the individual triumphs, the personal symphonies of success that our members experience every day.

So, let us embrace the untapped potential of the GLP-1's and the novel medications to come, not as a mere footnote in the annals of medical history, but as a groundbreaking chapter in the epic saga of human well-being.

Together, we'll compose a future where healthcare isn't just about surviving; it's about thriving in a world humming with possibility. Onward, to a future resounding with hope and harmony!

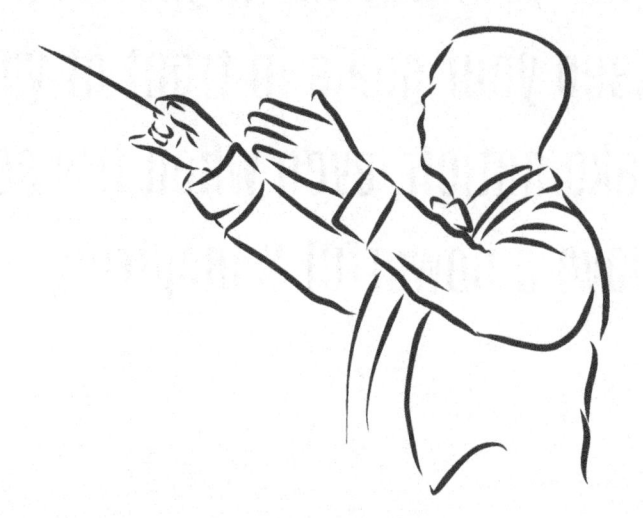

8 HABITS FOR SUCCESS

01. Read every day.
02. Focus on high-level tasks.
03. Make your health a priority.
04. Learn from people you admire.
05. Plan your day the night before.
06. Keep your goals in front of you.
07. Take action, even when it's scary.
08. Have a powerful & inspiring "why".

The SimpleMD® Manifesto

We believe wisdom is strength and simple is strong. We stand for truth, access and peace. We believe that science and technology can be a part of customized solutions that can work for us rather than against us. We believe in health and wellness as a lifestyle that starts with easy wins that become positive forward momentum that evolves into unstoppable habits.

We prioritize sustainable success over the fastest process. We know the time is right for you to start and that with our help results are withing your reach. We know you have friends and family that love you and want you around for years to come. We will fight against what hurts you, confuses you and misleads you from making your best life.

We dare to do it right. We dare to live long and we will love the journey as much as the destination.

Join us.

Start today.

Prepare for tomorrow.

Break free now.

Dr. Soffer

SimpleMD.com

Online Resources

www.SimpleMD.com

www.SimpleMDBook.com

Reading List

For Inspiration and Education

1. *Outlive* by Peter Attia, MD

2. *Do Hard Things* by Steve Magness

3. *Fitter. Calmer. Stronger.* by Ellie Goulding

4. *The Mind Gut Connection* by Emeran Mayer, MD

5. *Young Forever* by Mark Hyman, MD

6. *Make Your Bed* by Admiral William H. McRaven

7. *If Our Bodies Could Talk* by James Hamblin, MD

8. *Move* by Caroline Williams

9. *The Power of Self-Discipline* by Peter Hollins

10. *The Fitness Mindset* by Brian Keane

Online Resources

Made in the USA
Las Vegas, NV
11 October 2023